Beautifully Created

In *Beautifully Created*, Andrea Stephens shows you that you are God's masterpiece... a work of art. In this positive, practical book, she teaches you how to have a glowing beauty that radiates from within. A former fashion model, Andrea provides step-by-step techniques, full-color photographs, illustrations, and insightful projects, which will help you create your own style. You'll find solutions for problem areas and advice for making the most of what God has given you. This book includes guidelines for:

- sensational skin
- healthy self-image
- perfect posture
- model-style makeup
- building a better body
- nurturing hands and nails
- a wardrobe that works
- inner beauty... the essential for outer beauty

God loves you just as you are! Appreciate yourself because you are *Beautifully Created*.

Beautifully Created

Andrea Stephens

Fleming H. Revell Company
Old Tappan, New Jersey

Unless otherwise identified, Scripture quotations are from the New American Standard Bible, © The Lockman Foundation 1960, 1962, 1963, 1968, 1971, 1972, 1973, 1975, 1977.

Scripture quotations identified AMP are from AMPLIFIED BIBLE, OLD TESTAMENT, Copyright 1962, 1964 by Zondervan Publishing House, and are used by permission.

Library of Congress Cataloging-in-Publication Data

Stephens, Andrea.
   Beautifully created.

   1. Beauty, Personal. 2. Adolescent girls—
Health and hygiene. 3. Self-perception. 4. Christian
life—1960–   . I. Title.
RA778.S799   1987   646.7′042   87-20533
ISBN 0-8007-1549-7

All rights reserved. No part of this publication may be reproduced, stored in a retrieval system, or transmitted in any form or by any means—electronic, mechanical, photocopy, recording, or any other—except for brief quotations in printed reviews, without the prior permission of the publishers.

Copyright © 1987 by Andrea Stephens
Published by the Fleming H. Revell Company
Old Tappan, New Jersey 07675

This book is dedicated to
every young woman who has ever secretly wished
she were someone else.
May the Lord reveal to your heart
that you truly are Beautifully Created.

CONTENTS

1
A HEALTHY SELF-IMAGE
The Road to a More Beautiful You   15

WHAT IS SELF-IMAGE ANYWAY?
SELF-IMAGE FROM OTHERS—EXPERIENCES—
CIRCUMSTANCES—PHYSICAL APPEARANCE •
IMPROVING YOUR SELF-IMAGE •
THE TOP TEN
SELF-IMAGE TIPS

2
VISUAL POISE
Developing a Graceful Manner   29

WHAT IS VISUAL POISE? • *WHAT DIFFERENCE*
DOES POSTURE MAKE? •
SIX POINTS TO PERFECT POSTURE •
POSTURE EXERCISES •
STANDING • *WALKING RIGHT* •
TURNING AROUND • *SITTING PRETTY* •
MANAGING STAIRS • *VISUAL GRACES—LOOKING*
GOOD! • *INNER VISUAL POISE*

CONTENTS

3
SENSATIONAL SKIN
Sensible Steps to Great-Looking Skin   46

SKIN TYPES • NOURISHING YOUR SKIN •
SKIN CARE—THE BASICS—THE SPECIFICS •
DIRECTIONAL CHART •
BREAKOUT • SUN AND SKIN •
PREVENTING PROBLEMS

4
MODEL STYLE MAKEUP
Techniques Every Teen Should Know   61

ENHANCING YOUR APPEARANCE •
THE NATURAL LOOK •
BUILDING A BASE • FACE SCULPTING • POWDERED
PERFECTION •
EXPRESSIVE EYES • CHEERY CHEEKS •
LOVELY LIPS • PRETTY AS A PICTURE

5
NUTRITION
Building a Better Body   75

THE FEARED FOUR-LETTER WORD—DIET •
HOW MUCH SHOULD I WEIGH? •
EATING HABITS • BALANCED FOOD PROGRAM •
DELICIOUS DESSERTS •
SENSIBLE SNACKS • WHAT TO AVOID •
CALORIE CONSCIOUSNESS •
WEIGHT GAIN—ADDING POUNDS •
WEIGHT LOSS—SUBTRACTING POUNDS •
THE WHYS BEHIND OUR EATING •
MY PERSONAL STORY •
EFFECTS OF DRUGS AND ALCOHOL •
FEEDING YOUR SPIRIT

CONTENTS

6
TOTAL FITNESS
Just for the Fun of It 91

AEROBIC EXERCISE • AEROBIC TIPS • NONAEROBIC EXERCISE • EXERCISE ATTIRE • MY EXERCISE AUTOBIOGRAPHY • EXERCISING YOUR FAITH

7
HAIR HAPPENINGS
Styles That Give You Style 116

BASIC CARE • A CUT ABOVE • THE RIGHT STYLE FOR YOU • TYPES OF CUTS AND TERMS • SPECIAL EFFECTS • TOOLS AND TECHNIQUES • SIMPLE STYLES—SUPER LOOKS • TRICKS AND TIPS • WHAT AFFECTS HAIR? • THE ONE WHO CARES ABOUT YOUR HAIR

8
HANDS AND NAILS
Nurtured to Perfection 139

WHAT YOU WILL NEED • MANICURE MAGIC • PATCHING A NAIL—THE PAINLESS WAY • INSTANT NAILS • BEAUTY TIPS FOR NAILS • HELPING HANDS • BEAUTY TIPS FOR HANDS • FANCY FEET

9
DAZZLE YOURSELF WITH COLOR
Discovering Your Season and Colors 147

UNDERSTANDING THE SEASONS • ANY COLOR, ACCURATE SHADE • IDENTIFYING YOUR SEASON • COLOR AND YOUR WARDROBE • COLOR AND YOUR FIGURE • MOOD, IMPACT, DECORATING • COLOR AND THE COLOR WHEEL

CONTENTS

10
FUNCTIONING FASHION
A Wardrobe That Works   156

STYLES—CLASSICS AND FADS • BEING A SMART SHOPPER • DRESSING YOUR FIGURE • FABRICS AFFECT YOUR FIGURE, TOO • ORGANIZING YOUR WARDROBE • PIECING THE PUZZLE TOGETHER • BASIC SURVIVAL WARDROBE FOR TEENS • ACCESSORIES—AN ADDITIONAL TOUCH • PROPER CARE FOR LONG-LASTING WEAR • DRESSED OUTSIDE—DRESSED INSIDE • PUTTING IT ALL TOGETHER

11
DELICATE DETAILS
The Secrets of Personal Grooming   180

UNDERGARMENTS • MOUTH MATTERS • A BATH A DAY KEEPS THE ODOR AWAY • PUT AN END TO ROUGH SKIN • BATH TIME EXTRAS • AFTER-BATH PAMPERING—IT DOES A BODY GOOD • UNDERARM PROTECTION • REMOVING UNWANTED HAIR • HEAVENLY SCENT

12
INNER BEAUTY
Beauty Through and Through   187

WHAT IS INNER BEAUTY? • BUILDING BLOCKS TO INNER BEAUTY • UNDER CONSTRUCTION • BEHOLDING HIS BEAUTY • BEAUTY TAKES TIME

SELF-IMAGE PROGRESS REPORT   198

INDEX   201

ACKNOWLEDGMENTS

I always flipped right past the acknowledgments page of a book, thinking, *Oh brother, here come all the thank yous to everybody and his brother, grandmother, neighbor, mailman, dog, pet turtle, and God.*

Well, now I have a new appreciation for this special page. I have learned that you can't write a book totally by yourself. You need others. The Lord provided the talented people needed to pull this book together, and they just can't go unrecognized.

So, I *am* going to thank everybody and his brother and so on—except I'm not going to thank my pet turtle because I don't have one.

A big hug and grateful thank you to:

Carol Lacy, for your expertise, guidance, and love. You made this happen.

Barbra Minar, for reading, pre-editing, and adding motherly advice.

Carol Mulker, for diligently typing and retyping—always with a smile.

Lizbeth Kyle, for your wonderful illustrations.

Leslie Holtzman, for your creative photography skills.

Lisa Marie Welton, for your hairstyling and techniques.

ACKNOWLEDGMENTS

Jennifer Hopson, for filling in with last-minute illustrations.

Kim, Kara, Nicole, Amy, Jenni, Maili, Sally, and LaBelle models Seanna and Teresa, for gracing these pages with your smiling faces.

Susan Halme, for graciously lending me clothes and accessories from Elna's Dress Shop and The Courtyard.

Bill Stephens, for being an understanding husband.

Special thanks to my parents and family, those who previewed this manuscript, and those who had me on their prayer lists!

And of course, the Lord, for giving me a vision and showing me how to make it happen. You are faithful.

Beautifully Created

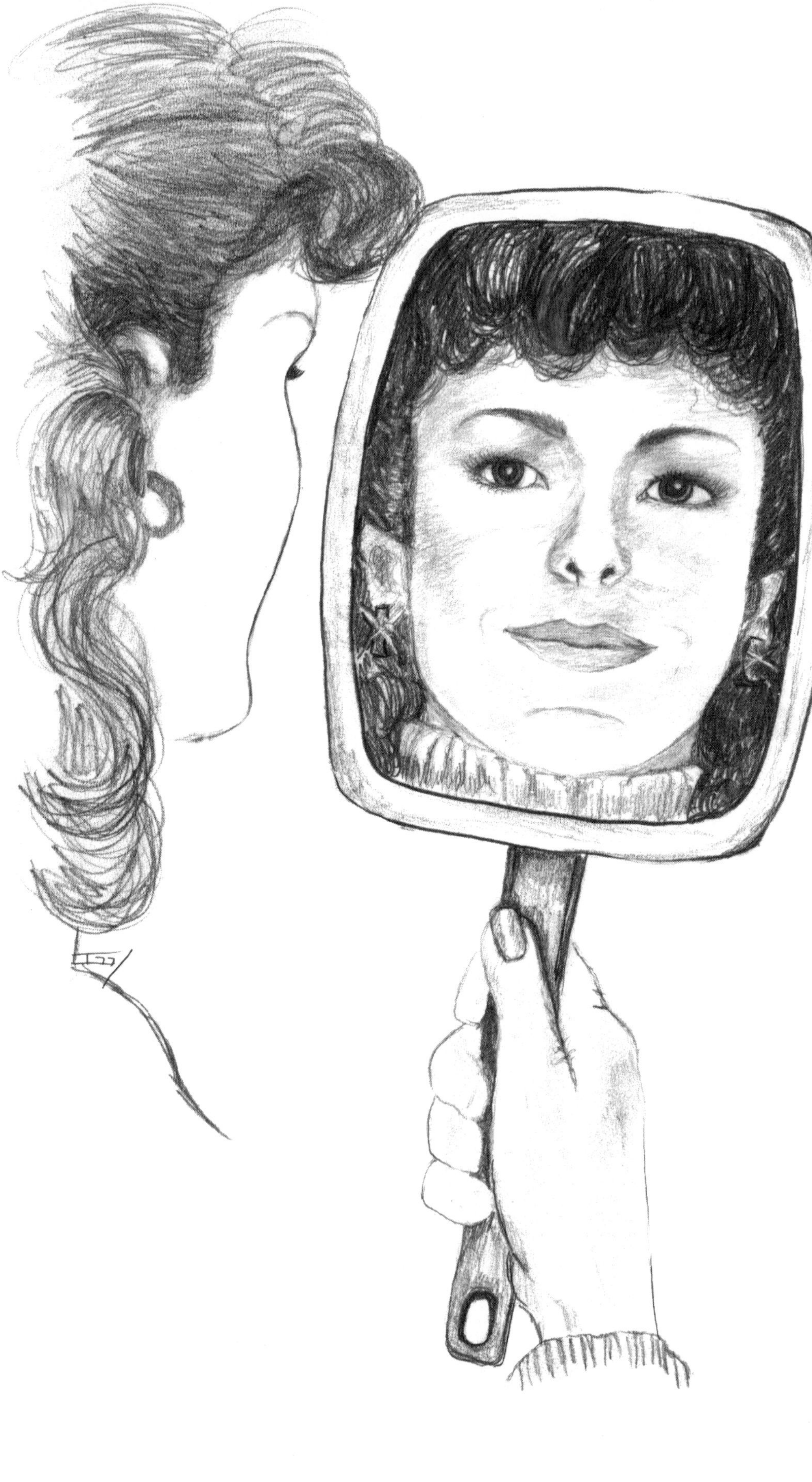

1 A HEALTHY SELF-IMAGE
The Road to a More Beautiful You

Did you know that there is a weird disease among teenagers that's spreading outrageously fast? Oh, it's not a picky disease—it doesn't care who it attacks! You can be rich or poor, sophisticated or cutesy, pudgy or skinny, talented, unskilled, intelligent, famous or unknown. You can live on the east or west coast, on a mountaintop or in a valley, Beverly Hills or the New York City ghetto. It can track you down wherever you are!

The symptoms of this outrageous yet all-too-common disease show up in many ways: your reaction to a pimple smack dab in the middle of your forehead that feels like Mount St. Helens; a feeling that your wardrobe is dull instead of dashing; realizing that being taller than all the boys you know or shorter than your little sister seriously bugs you. Still other symptoms might be the frustration you sense when you are getting a 2.5 grade point average while your brother or sister always pulls through with a 4.0. Perhaps not having a close friend or not liking where you live or the school you go to is your symptom. More serious symptoms could be brought on by a broken home or the loss of a loved one or a pet. Or the ultimate symptom, complete despair—your hair frizzed out just before that all-important, once-a-year event: school pictures.

This disease can cause its victims to act in strange and unaccountable ways. Some withdraw and become shy around their friends. Others push to be overly outgoing—the class loudmouth. They act in these ways hoping no one will notice that they have the disease.

The ultimate result of the disease is total self-dislike, a belief that you have no value, nothing to contribute to life. Everything you do is wrong. *Oh,* you think, *if only I could be someone else!*

Do you know anyone with these symptoms? Perhaps you have met someone who has this disease. Maybe you have even discovered a few symptoms in yourself. Oooh, scary!

Have you guessed the disease yet? It's not measles or chicken pox! Right! This crummy, life-robbing disease is a *low self-image.*

Almost every teenager I know—especially girls—at some time struggles with a low self-image. They feel as if they just don't measure up and aren't as good as others.

Is there a cure? Yes! The cure is to discover who you are and how you fit into your Creator's plan. To understand how uniquely you have been created, and that there has never been—and never will be—anyone exactly like you, the gifts and talents you have, and the fact that God loves you so much, no matter what, will lead you to a healthy recovery from this dreadful disease.

Self-image is an important topic to deal with. Your self-image can be your best friend or your worst enemy. It will either limit you or allow you to grow. How you see yourself, how you think others see you, and the way you feel about yourself affect almost everything you do and every relationship you are in. In fact, having a self-image that is too high or too low stops you from seeing yourself clearly. A good self-image does not come from what you have or what you look like but from accepting yourself the way God made you and sees you—beautiful, forgiven, lovable, worthy, and a winner! Watch how the Holy Spirit will take you, just as you give yourself to Him, and mold you into the royal image God has in mind for you.

If you currently have a low self-image, this next statement might be hard for you to believe, but it's true: God loves you just the way He designed you! And He wants *you* to love you also! He wants you to see yourself as the valuable young woman He has made you to be: loving, believing in, and being yourself. A good self-image is the first priority in developing a more beautiful you. That's what this book is about: first, to accept yourself as you are—even though you think you are not the "ideal," and second, to discover how to take what you are and enhance it so that you make the most of what God has given you.

In her book *The American Look,* well-known actress Jaclyn Smith says, "You have to be sincerely happy with and interested in being you for anyone's beauty advice to be of value."

Are you interested in you? I hope so. Let's take a close look at your self-image so you can understand it better. Then we will make changes where they are needed. This is the first step down the road to a beautiful you!

What Is Self-Image Anyway?

The word *self* refers to you. The real person deep inside. Image means a mental picture, thought, idea, and impression. So, self-image is the picture you have in your mind; the thought, idea, and impression you have of you! It is the way you see yourself and how you feel about yourself. Good or bad, everyone has a self-image.

Many factors form your self-image. Some you have control over; others you don't. The point to remember as you discover the factors that have formed your self-image is that self-image is changeable.

Self-Image From Others

What a beautiful day! Ginny felt good. Everything had gone well all day at school. She shifted the load of books she was carrying and suddenly lost her grip on them. They scattered all over the sidewalk just as a carload of guys drove by. One of them leaned out the window and shouted, "Klutz!" Immediately everything changed. Ginny turned bright red with embarrassment. Behind her, her best friend saw what happened and caught up with her. "Way to go, clumsy," she teased. "You need charm school!" That little incident planted a seed in Ginny's mind: *I'm a klutz. I'm stupid and clumsy and I look silly.*

Like Ginny, most of us draw conclusions about who we are and what our value is by gathering information about ourselves from others. When a parent walks out on your family, when a boyfriend suddenly breaks up with you without an explanation, or when a close friend no longer speaks to you, your self-image is affected. Parents, brothers and sisters, friends, peers, teachers, coaches, employers, youth workers—all of these people play a part in the way you see yourself. How you interpret the statements they make about you and the way they act and react toward you will cause you to form a mental picture of yourself. This is a natural process. But we must be selective in this process.

Becoming Someone You're Not

Accepting evaluations from others of who you are may make you act the way you think *they* want you to act. We all know people who try to be someone they are not. Why would anyone try to be what others think they should be? The answer to this question comes from a need that all of us have: to be loved and accepted for who we are. We want to feel that we are okay and approved of. Sometimes we'll even compromise what we believe, just to be accepted. Who wants to be different or a misfit? No one wants to feel as if they don't fit in. So, we try to please others by being what they want us to be.

But wait—is that really a good exchange? Doesn't that mean we are second best? Yes! Being what others want you to be will always make you second best. You can be yourself better than anyone else can. Oh sure, choosing to be what others want you to be might bring temporary acceptance, but it's not the real thing. The real you is best. Why settle for second when you can be tops?

Before you accept what others say about you as fact, ask yourself these questions:

1. Who is the person giving his or her opinion of you?
2. What value or position does he or she hold in your life?
3. Is this person a relative, an acquaintance, a buddy, a casual friend, or a close friend?

Your relationship to the person will affect how seriously you take his or her opinion. A close friend's comments will count more than those of an acquaintance! But even friends tease a lot, and sometimes their comments need to be taken lightly. After all, they are coping with self-image also. Choosing friends who are honest, trustworthy, dependable, and most of all, caring Christians, may minimize hurtful teasing.

Parents, like friends, tend to make comments about us that we take to heart. Sometimes parents are funny creatures! They drop hints or make direct statements that we take very personally. They don't do this purposely to hurt our feelings. They really love us very much and do want what is best for us. Unfortunately, when they correct us in these ways, their love is not always the message we pick up. Nevertheless, the Bible says we are to love and obey our parents, forgiving them even when their words sting.

Your self-image must be built on solid ground, not on the opinions of others. So, be sure that what you believe about yourself is accurate. Your self-image is counting on you!

Dreams of the Heart—Promoted or Pounced On?

When I was a teenager, I had a strong desire to model. I got involved with fashion shows, learned how to apply makeup properly, and like many other girls, daydreamed about having my picture taken for the cover of *Seventeen*. When I was a senior in high school, I secretly sent a copy of my graduation picture to a top modeling agency. After several weeks, a response arrived. The agency sent back my picture with the reply that I would never be a model and should look into another career. The agency executives informed me that they were experts in the modeling field. I could seek the advice of others, but I would be wasting my time. I could not be a model.

Right then I had a decision to make. I could either believe what those "experts" said or stick with my inner feeling that I could be a model. I was determined to hang in there. I didn't let their opinion determine how I felt about myself.

Less than two years later I was offered a modeling contract by Wilhelmina herself of Wilhelmina Models, Inc. Off I moved to New York. I will be the first to admit that I am certainly no Christie Brinkley, but I have had several exciting national modeling jobs and the opportunity to meet many well-known people. I am glad I decided not to accept the "expert" advice from the other agency.

When you let others' opinions of you form your self-image, it may limit you in fulfilling the desires of your heart. It doesn't matter what they think. If *you* can see yourself fulfilling your secret dream, then you are well on your way to doing it! Why let others limit you? Besides, you have an unlimited God on your side!

Limitations—Some Real, Some Imagined

I realize that if I were five feet, three inches tall, the idea of modeling would have been unrealistic. If your secret dreams and inner desires are realistic, go for them. There are really only a few things that might limit you in doing and becoming all you see yourself becoming. For instance, *you may be physically limited*. Girls can't be guys because they are girls! Or, if you are four feet, eight inches tall, you probably won't be a star basketball player!

Perhaps you have a physical handicap. This may restrict you in some ways, but it may also steer you to the specific plan God has for your life.

As a teenager, Joni Eareckson Tada was left a quadriplegic and confined to a wheelchair after a diving accident. She could have refused to try to make something out of her life with what she had left, but she didn't. Through many trials and many tears, Joni developed two talents with the part of her not affected by the accident. She is well known for the drawings she does with a pencil in her mouth, and she has released several record albums. With God's help, it is possible to make the most of your life. He has a plan for each of us.

Lack of knowledge can also limit you. Usually this is temporary. Many people do not attempt to do things they have never learned to do. I can't speak Spanish but that's because I have never been taught. It is not a matter of being stupid or limited, it's because I have never taken the time to learn. The Bible tells us in Proverbs 10:14 that people who are wise store up or grow in knowledge. Learning is very important. Some kids don't like school, or at least don't take it very seriously. I hope you are wise enough to know how valuable learning really is. You don't have to let lack of knowledge limit you.

Doubt is the most effective limiter of all! If you don't think you can, then you can't. Believe in your heart you can do it! Why? Because from your heart you will get the strength to complete the task that is facing you. Many times in the Scriptures we are encouraged to be believers, not doubters. Jesus referred to His disciples as men of little faith. He wants us to be of BIG faith. One of the disciples, Thomas, better known as "Doubting Thomas," was told by Jesus, "Stop your doubting and believe." We need to understand that what the angel told Mary, Mother of Jesus, is true: "Nothing will be impossible with God" (Luke 1:37). Believing in yourself and in God is the key to overcoming doubt.

Oh Lord, You Want Me to *What?*

There is one other thing Christians need to take into consideration: Perhaps what you want for yourself isn't what God has planned for your life. Oh, you can go ahead with your plans, disregarding what God wants for you. But one day you'll wake up and say, "I've been foolish! Look at the time I've wasted going my own way."

While I was modeling in New York, I really wanted a successful career. Modeling seems glamorous and exciting, but with it comes many challenges. I was constantly making value judgments. I always wanted to do what was right and pleasing to the Lord. Sometimes I did. Sometimes I didn't. But, thank the Lord, He is forgiving! After a year or so, I felt unfulfilled in my modeling pursuit and I stopped going my way long enough to sense that God had something else in mind for me. So, I gradually began to change my way and to follow more closely the Lord's plan for my life. I have never regretted it for a minute, and you won't either. Doing what God wants is not always easy, but it is always worth it. God rewards us in His own special way for following His plans. Our heavenly Father loves us so much and wants what is best for us.

Self-Image From Experiences

Even though she had just turned seventeen, Maggie was given a lot of responsibility in her job as assistant manager of Kimby Toy Store. Every night she was to count the money in the cash register, then leave one hundred dollars in the register and deposit the rest at the bank's night deposit box. But one night she had a problem. She lost the deposit key. She usually kept it handy in her wallet, but it wasn't there.

She couldn't reach her manager, so Maggie decided the best thing to do was to take the money home. She would call the manager in the morning and explain where the money was. But she forgot to call.

At school the next day, during third period, Maggie was abruptly removed from class because there was an emergency phone call for her. It was her manager at the toy store. He was irate. Where was the money? How could she forget to call him? Why was she so irresponsible? Could she really be trusted?

Maggie was crushed. She had thought taking the money with her was the safest thing to do. She thought she was being responsible. The manager tried to make her feel lousy about herself. Of course, it was her fault she had not called him. But Maggie knew that, except for that oversight, she had acted in the best way.

You often draw conclusions about who you are from your own experiences. Sometimes these conclusions are right, sometimes wrong. This depends on how you view the experience. Maggie could have decided she was careless and untrustworthy, but she didn't. Sure, she had made a mistake, but that didn't make her a bad person.

There will, of course, be times when you fail, disobey, or just plain mess up. We fall short of our own expectations, others' expectations of us, and even God's expectations. Everyone has times when they fail a test, lose a game, miss an appointment, lie, break a promise, snap at their parents, or neglect their prayer time with the Lord. Some of these not-so-hot experiences are your own responsibility—like making the wrong decision when you knew the right thing to do. Other experiences are caused by other people. These you have less control over.

Yet, you can make the most of every experience you have. Here's how!

First, stop and examine yourself, so you know when you need to make some positive changes in the things you are doing. This will help make more positive the experiences *you* are responsible for.

Second, forgive yourself for your failures and shortcomings. Equally important to forgiving yourself is forgetting these bad experiences. Forgiving and forgetting go hand in hand. If you think you have forgiven yourself for something, but continue to remind yourself of it over and over, have you really forgiven yourself? Probably not!

God forgives you and forgets your sins when you sincerely ask Him to. The Bible says He doesn't remember your sins anymore. He puts your sins as far as the East is from the West—and the East and West never meet! God is not up in heaven with a tally board of everything you have ever done wrong. He is not holding anything against you once you have asked His forgiveness. Do what Paul, a servant of Jesus, did. He said he forgot the past and looked toward the future.

Third, just as important as forgiving yourself is forgiving those who have caused you to have bad experiences. I know this is very hard. In fact, it doesn't even seem fair. But the Lord tells us it's our responsibility to forgive. Why do you think Jesus says we must forgive others? There are two main reasons: One, so that in turn, God will forgive us our wrongdoings. Two, so that we will once again be free to love those people who have hurt us. God doesn't want us to be broken people or to have broken relationships.

Sometimes you don't think the hurt others have caused you will ever go away, but your Father God can touch you with His healing power and make you whole. To heal you spiritually, emotionally, and physically is one of the reasons Jesus died for us. Ask Him to heal your hurt. I know He will.

Successful experiences, failing experiences, good experiences, bad experiences . . . they all team up to help shape you into God's best!

Self-Image From Circumstances

In addition to the opinions of others and your experiences, your circumstances may affect the way you feel about yourself. Several years ago I attended a meeting at a counseling center for unwed teenage mothers. The goal of the center was to make it possible for girls to have their babies rather than let them think abortion was the only solution. As the close of the meeting drew near, a woman in her mid-twenties stood and walked to the front of the room. In a shy yet strong voice, she told us her story.

"My mother became pregnant as a teenager and was unmarried. She felt alone, embarrassed, and full of shame. She thought the only way out was to abort the tiny person growing inside of her. But just before she was about to carry through with her plans, the Lord sent a woman into her life whom she was able to trust and with whom she could share the crisis she was facing. This special woman made the way possible for my mother to do what she really wanted to do—give birth to her baby. That baby was me."

The young woman standing before us did not choose to be born into a situation that gave her no family, no sense of belonging, and years of wondering why her real father didn't want her. These were circumstances in her life she had no control over. And they were unchangeable. But she was given the greatest gift: life.

You can choose to accept or reject the circumstances in your life that are unchangeable. Your parents, your brothers and sisters, your birth position in your family, your race, your skin color, and the fact that you are a female, are all circumstances you were born into which you can't change. Whether or not you accept these circumstances will have an effect on your self-image.

Realizing that each of your unchangeable circumstances has been given to you for a purpose will help you be open to accepting them. Your life—all it is and all it isn't—is God's gift to you; what you do with it is your gift to God. Since the Bible says that God is for you, who or what can work against you? Your life's circumstances are not meant to work against you. Like the young woman we just met, see how you can take what you have been given and make something good out of it. Let your circumstances help build up your self-image rather than get you down.

Self-Image From Physical Appearance

Another thing that influences your self-image is your physical appearance. If you are like the many teenage girls I know, you have some physical features you would be much happier without! Everyone I know has something she would trade in with no hesitation. Oh, if only that were possible!

We live in a society that says if you don't like what you look like, change it! Nose too long? Get it shortened. Eyes not green enough? Colored contacts will fix that. Hair won't curl? Perm it. Hair won't straighten? Straighten it. The signs of aging getting to you? Visit your local plastic surgeon for a face-lift! Not happy with your bust line? Two thousand dollars will get you a new one. Don't want brown hair? Become a blonde—directly from a bottle! Nails refuse to grow? Slap on some acrylic ones! The list goes on and on.

Certainly all of these things are not wrong, but they are proof that the majority of people today have a hard time accepting their given physical appearance. And why wouldn't they? There is so much emphasis on physical beauty in the American culture. Every billboard and magazine cover sends us the same message. Surely you need an oval face, high cheekbones, perfectly straight white teeth, bouncing hair, flawless skin, and weigh not an ounce over 110 pounds, to be accepted. Right? WRONG! Less than 1 percent of the world's population has these combined characteristics. Almost every picture-perfect face you see in print has been airbrushed to look flawless!

It is difficult to escape the pressure of trying to look like a cover girl in order to gain self-acceptance and the attention of others. Women, and especially teens, end up believing in these beauty standards that really are impossible to achieve. Then when we compare our own appearance to these standards, what happens? We don't measure up. But how could we? It is a false image we are comparing ourselves to. Yet we feel like going through life with paper bags over our heads!

It is my guess that none of you had a thing to do with the way you look. While you were still inside your mother, did she call you up on the umbilical cord to ask you what you wanted to look like? Did anyone let you put in special requests before you were designed? I know I didn't get that chance. I would have asked to be one and a half inches taller and to have fewer freckles!

Liking Your Looks

Why do some girls have such a tough time accepting their physical appearance? One reason may be that all of us have been teased about our looks. It begins when we are children. "Where did you get all those freckles?" "Boy, you're a skinny little thing. Don't you ever eat?" Or, "I'll bet your mother never has leftovers at your house." People can be thoughtless when it comes to identifying your differences. Of course they always pick a feature you can't help! Big noses are referred to as ski slopes, and oversized ears are often called Dumbo ears. What about Bozo Hair, Four Eyes, and Metal

Mouth? Any of these sound familiar? I was continually called Bird Legs as a kid. So my legs were skinny. No fault of mine!

Nicknames are often unfair. They can hurt us more than others realize, and more than we care to show. I call them "kicknames" because that is exactly what they do! These seemingly playful put-downs, when connected to your physical appearance, can make you question your looks.

Please don't take someone's sorry sense of humor to heart! People who tease and put others down are usually struggling with their own self-acceptance. Sometimes they actually think their comments are cute, but it is interpreted by you as faultfinding.

The Word of God tells us in Ephesians 4:29 that we are to edify one another. *Edify* means to build up. We are to build each other up, not put each other down! Do you build up or put down those around you? And what about yourself? This principle applies to the things you say to yourself as well. Stop insulting yourself and others. You are a precious person. Build yourself and others up in the Lord.

Lack of Attention

Not getting enough attention may be another reason for not liking your appearance. Some kids feel the whole world is ignoring them, so they must be ugly! Ever sit home on a Saturday night without a date, convincing yourself that you are not as cute as Suzy Smoozy, who always has a date? Not getting the attention you need or want may have nothing to do with your looks. However, the effect will be the same if you think it does. Look at the girl who gets attention only because she looks great. Does anyone take her seriously as a person? She's just good to look at and makes the guys who go with her look good. (Remember, guys have a self-image problem, too!) Being liked for who you are on the inside is far more important. As Christians we have an extra bonus when it comes to attention. We have a Lord who is always available and ready to give us His full love and attention. We matter to Him! He cares how we feel.

God's Design for You

Maybe you struggle with your looks because you don't truly understand that God is your Designer. He created the first man and woman, and in describing how He made them, He said, "It is very good." Then He said to multiply. His creation is still "good"; differences in our appearances are good. Don't you think He is capable of bringing out your best, of emphasizing *your* uniqueness? Everything God creates has value. Everything He creates is beautiful. This includes you! God sees you as beautiful. The Lord wants you to know in your heart that He has placed His stamp of approval on you.

You are much more than just a little bit of your mother and a little bit of your father mixed together. Your parents had a lot to do with your appearance, but God knew who you would be long before you were born. You were God's idea!

In the very first book of the Bible, Genesis, God says He made us in His image and His likeness. We are made like Him. What an honor! Of all the creatures He created, God chose *us* to be like Him.

The Bible says it was God's hands

that fashioned you and made you. You are handmade! Psalms 139:13, 14 tells you that God formed your inward parts and wove you while you were still growing inside your mother. Look very closely at a weaving and you will notice each strand of yarn is placed very carefully to create the design the artist wanted. This is the same kind of care and planning God used to make you. The passage goes on to say that you are fearfully and wonderfully made. The word *fearfully* means with honor and respect, not that God was afraid when He made you. You are wonderfully made. Verse 15 says that your frame—your bone structure—is uniquely yours. You must be pretty important.

Most amazing of all, the Bible tells you in Genesis 2:7 that it is God's very breath that gave Adam, the first human, life. That creation cycle continues today. God's breath has given *you* life.

Wow! You *are* God-created. Is there any question left in your mind? You are a unique creation, handcrafted by the Master Designer. There's no stamp on you that says MADE IN AMERICA. It says MADE IN HEAVEN! The Lord made you beautiful, and He loves how He made you. He sees you through eyes of love.

Defects or Details?

"But wait," you say, "what about the things *I* don't like about my appearance? What about the marks and shapes I think are mistakes or flaws?" Here is the answer: These things are far from flaws; they are the intricate details on your individual appearance that make you *one-of-a-kind*. There is no one else like you. No one can take your place. I'm so glad God didn't have just one or two "people" molds. If we all looked alike, life would be much less exciting!

The details of your appearance do not make you different in a negative sense. They make you special. You have a certain look that sets you apart from all others. Accepting this will help you achieve God's purpose for your life.

Feelings of dislike toward your appearance are common. No need to feel guilty! In fact, the Bible even talks about it. Romans 9:20 says, "How can the clay say to the potter, 'Why have you made me this way?' " (*See* Today's English Version—Good News Bible.) Have you ever asked God this question? It may take some time to understand, but you are the clay in the hands of the Potter, God. He is making you the way that pleases Him and fits into the plan He has for your life. You may not understand that plan right now, but you will. Try asking God what He has in store for your life. I promise His answer will bless you!

Beware! Don't compare your appearance with the appearance of others, especially in specific areas you can't change. Comparing only leads to one of two conclusions: (1) you are better than so-and-so, or (2) you are not as good as so-and-so. Both of these attitudes are wrong. The first one is prideful and conceited. The second one makes you feel inferior—as if you don't measure up. I'll let you in on a little secret. Many times in your life you will meet people you think are more attractive than you are, and you will meet others you think are less attractive. Remembering that *in God's eyes all of us are equally beautiful* will help you not to compare.

You can develop a healthy self-image by accepting God's design for you. Which will you choose to believe—the world's beauty standards or God's?

Improving Your Self-Image

We have looked at four major influences in the development of your self-image: *others, experiences, circumstances,* and *physical appearance.* Therefore, you have already learned four ways to improve your self-image: First, evaluate the things others are saying before you accept them as fact. Second, learn from unsuccessful experiences and be forgiving toward yourself and others. Third, accept the circumstances in your life that you can't change. Fourth, learn to love God's design for your physical appearance. Each of these will give you a good start on improving your self-image.

The girls who have taken my Beautifully Created course have come up with a few more tips I know you will find helpful. Try these to get an image boost.

The Top Ten Self-Image Tips

1. Get a good mental picture of the new image you want, and grow into it. Remember that self-image means the picture, thoughts, ideas, and impressions you have of you.

2. Set goals. Include several short goals you can reach quickly and with some ease. This will build your success rate and make you feel as if you are getting somewhere. This is a real confidence builder. Be sure your goals are big enough to include God's help.

3. Be yourself. Get excited about being unique. Step out and be a leader. This will help others be themselves also.

4. Discover your natural talents and gifts. What things come naturally to you? These are probably from God. Sports, music, working with children, organizing, art—the list goes on. Concentrate on your special talents.

5. Write a list of twenty-five good things about yourself. You may have to think hard, but I know you can do it! If you also discover some not-so-hot things about yourself, such as character traits that you can change, write them down also, and see how you can improve so you can get those traits over on the list of good things.

6. Surround yourself with honest and dependable Christian friends, those who make you feel good about who you are. Encourage one another to be your best.

7. Learn a new subject or hobby. Expand yourself!

8. Read God's Word daily. You can always find a message of love and hope when you need it. The more you read, the more you will realize that you can do all things with Jesus!

9. Try some quick picker-uppers! Do something special for someone else. This will work wonders for liking yourself better. Wear a new hairstyle or outfit. Place a fresh-cut flower in a vase on your bed stand. Take a nice long bubble bath. Oh, what fun!

10. Believe in yourself. God has begun a good thing in you and He will complete it!

Having a healthy and clear image of who you are is truly the beginning of a beautiful you. Beauty begins on the inside, then shines outward.

Now that you are well on your way to a better-looking self-image, let's get started on enhancing your outer image.

A HEALTHY SELF-IMAGE

Project Page

1. Having a low self-image is a common disease. Do you know anyone who suffers from this illness? List some symptoms of a low self-image. _____
   _____
   _____
   _____

2. Have you ever wished you could be someone else? Who would you be? Why? _____
   _____
   _____
   _____

3. Do you ever feel as if you don't quite measure up to most people? Read 2 Corinthians 10:15. What does this verse tell you about comparing yourself with others? _____
   _____
   _____
   _____

4. Why do you think it's hard for people to believe God loves them just the way He designed them? _____
   _____
   _____
   _____

5. Describe how you see yourself right now. What do you think has influenced this image? _____
   _____
   _____
   _____

6. Like Ginny, we all draw conclusions about ourselves from what others say about us and to us. Think of a time when someone said something about you and you took it to heart. How did it affect your self-image? _____
   _____
   _____
   _____

7. Have you ever tried to be what someone else wanted you to be? What happened?

8. What are the secret dreams of your heart? What or who is stopping you from fulfilling them?

9. Of the three limiters—physical, knowledge, doubt—which one hinders you most often?

10. List three not-so-hot experiences you have had. How did your reactions to these experiences affect how you felt about yourself?

11. Is there a person you have been holding a grudge against? Ask God to help you to forgive the person, to heal your hurt, and then to help you be loving toward that person again.

12. Can you think of a negative experience in your life that God worked out for good?

13. What unchangeable circumstances in your life have been having a negative effect on your self-image? If you accept these circumstances and ask God to help you make the most of them, what changes might you expect?

14. If you have any physical features you would change if you could, list them here. Circle the ones that are unchangeable. Now pray and ask God to help you love every single part of your appearance—just the way He made you. _____
   _____
   _____
   _____

15. This next one takes courage! Look into a mirror and, one by one, thank God for every part of you. Remember Psalms 139:14: "I will give thanks to Thee, for I am fearfully and wonderfully made."

16. We all have been rejected at some time because of our appearance. Open your heart to Jesus and allow Him to heal the hurt you have felt. Write Him a letter expressing your feelings.

17. List five of your features that make you one-of-a-kind. _____
   _____
   _____
   _____
   _____

2 VISUAL POISE
Developing a Graceful Manner

"Me, graceful?" Could be! What does the word *graceful* mean to you? You may think of swans, flowing dancers, or even a quiet waterfall. *Graceful* means ease of movement; smooth, flowing, unforced gestures that come naturally. They may come naturally because of inborn coordination, or they may come naturally because a person has been taught correct movements and has practiced them to the point that they look natural and very graceful.

Have you ever noticed, though, that not everyone appears graceful in the same situations? You may feel graceful cruising on your bike but totally awkward in aerobic dance class. This is due to our individual God-given body types or frames, as Psalm 139 describes.

For example, let's look at Laura and Rachelle. Laura has a body that is athletically built. Her shoulders and hipbones are about the same width. This doesn't leave her with much of a waist. She has slightly large bones and is athletically coordinated. Rachelle, on the other hand, has a body that is fit more for dancing—a long trunk with slender features. She is rather small boned. Laura and Rachelle have different body types, but neither one has a "wrong" body type. However, in her own area, each girl appears more graceful than the other. Let's see how.

Laura and Rachelle had been best friends since junior high school. Through the years they had laughed together, shared their secret crushes, and helped each other during their high school years. Now, in their junior year, the girls were finding themselves involved in separate clubs, sports, and activities. Laura was deep into student council and student debate. More important, she was the star of the girls' softball team. She loved softball and was thrilled every time she broke a school record. Home runs were her favorite—seeing the ball fly into the stands far out of the reach of any other players, she smugly took her time running the bases. The cheers of the crowd always warmed her heart.

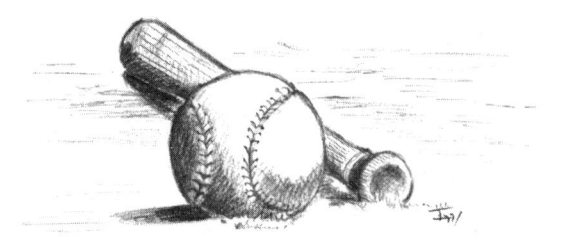

Rachelle was probably Laura's biggest fan. She never missed a game and always had a handful of confetti ready to toss into the air whenever Laura made a good play. She was amazed at the way Laura handled herself on the field.

Rachelle, however, found herself not on the baseball diamond but in a dance studio lined with glistening, full-length mirrors. She was a ballerina. Year after year, Rachelle had faithfully taken ballet lessons. She was very graceful by nature and had a high capacity for self-discipline. She had developed her talent far beyond most of her classmates. Rachelle dreamed of someday becoming a prima ballerina. Skilled moves, impressive choreography, fancy costumes, and a handsome partner were sure to be her future delight.

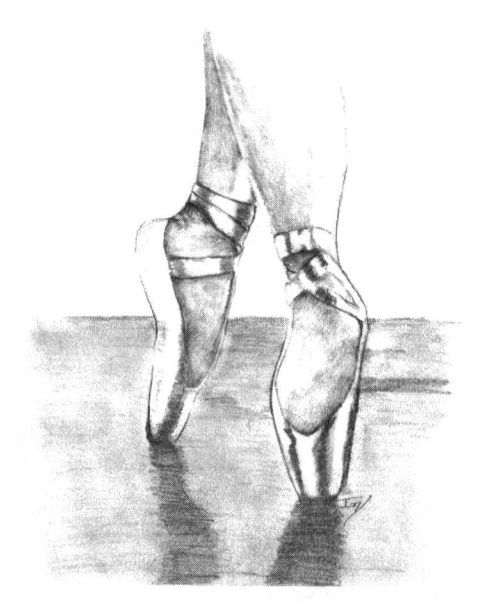

Laura, of course, made it to almost every one of Rachelle's recitals. She even sneaked in to see a few classes. She really admired Rachelle's flowing arm movements and effortless leaps. Laura never considered herself a graceful person, but to her, Rachelle was the ultimate in that area.

One day after school, the girls dropped by McDonald's to get diet Cokes and some fries. They were sharing the day's business and what they had going on that evening. Laura had softball practice, Rachelle had ballet rehearsal. Life seemed to have the girls involved in separate activities. This made them wonder if they really knew each other as well as they thought they did. They truly cared about their friendship and didn't want to drift apart just because of their different interests. Wouldn't it be fun, they thought, to trade places—just for one night—just for fun! They weren't sure they could pull it off, but they decided to give it a try.

What Laura and Rachelle learned about each other that night was unforgettable.

Laura was athletic, but she was no ballerina! Toe shoes and tights? *How does Rachelle do this?* she thought. Remembering all the times she had watched Rachelle gracefully tiptoe across the shiny wooden dance floor made her giggle at herself, trying desperately just to stand up!

Rachelle experienced a similar awakening as she made great attempts to match Laura's famous home runs. *Home run,* she thought, *I can hardly hit the ball!* Running the bases was no easy chore either. Why was second base so far away from first base? Rachelle admired Laura's ability even more now that she had stepped into her shoes. But she could hardly wait to get back into her toe shoes!

Are you getting the picture? Both Laura and Rachelle are unique young ladies. And both are graceful—Laura on the softball diamond and Rachelle in the dance studio.

Everyone is graceful in her own way. When you are taking a look at your own grace, be fair. Don't judge your gracefulness by someone else's standards. You are you. Discover the areas where being graceful comes naturally, and in situations where you feel less than comfortable, work on it!

Of course, gracefulness can be developed through knowing what moves appear graceful and through practice. Yes, *practice.* And self-discipline! It's almost like homework—you have to apply what you are learning before it makes any sense. So, apply what you are going to learn about visual poise.

What Is Visual Poise?

Let's define *visual poise: Visual*—what you can see with your eyes; outward appearance; that which can be seen. *Poise*—your composure or the way you carry yourself; the way you control your body movements. Putting it all together, visual poise is your outward control of your body movements. Sounds technical, doesn't it?

One benefit of developing graceful visual poise is that it will help you feel more confident in yourself and give a lift to your self-image.

Most important, it will help you relax. You won't have to be preoccupied with yourself, wondering whether or not you look good. Knowing that you look your best will give you the freedom to get your attention off yourself and onto others! This is true charm at its best—being as unselfconscious as possible!

In the beginning of the how-to's of visual poise, we need to start at the very core of what will be the foundation of your newly acquired gracefulness, and that is your posture.

What Difference Does Posture Make?

School physicals were never my favorite thing. Stuffy waiting rooms with 1930 waltz music playing was not my idea of a good time. Why these physicals were required, I was sure no one knew, but nevertheless, there I was for my 2:00 P.M. appointment. At least I was lucky enough to have a decent doctor—one who had an office full of photos of his four gorgeous sons! Somehow, stepping into Dr. Tullin's office was more like opening a *GQ* magazine than entering a cold, sterile examining room.

Dr. Tullin had a very gentle manner about him that I greatly appreciated when it came time to poke, push, and prod. He was also an honest man. After my physical was complete, Dr. T asked me to stand in front of the mirror above his sink. He turned me sideways and had me take a good look at myself. Slumped shoulders and a slightly rounded spine stared back at me from the mirror.

It was obvious. I was a young girl growing tall, and I wasn't quite sure how to handle myself.

The doctor proceeded to share with me the benefits of good posture and the confidence I could display through standing up straight and accepting my changing appearance. His words of wisdom really touched my heart, so I took his advice. Little did I know that that experience at the doctor's office was going to be a determining factor in my appearance.

Rarely do you see a model with bad posture. In fact, the most confident and successful people have already mastered the art of visual poise, especially posture.

Posture is best defined as the positioning of your body structure, or more simply, body alignment. Your posture is very important. Whether or not you realize it, your posture gives messages to others about who you are and how you feel about yourself. Your posture talks!

I'll describe three different types of posture and you write down your first impression of each.

First, we have Susy. She walks into a room with her head down, barely glancing around. Her shoulders are rounded and her neck leans forward. She is wearing an oversized flannel shirt and well-worn jeans.

Your impression is:

_____
_____
_____
_____

Second is Angela. Angela just can't be missed! Bouncing about the cafeteria, her neck and head are so far up that you are sure something's going to break! Angela carries her shoulders back *too* well, which leaves her chest held high and hard to miss. Angela usually has on the latest fashions and would not think of being caught without her makeup and hair totally perfect.

Your impression is:

_____
_____
_____
_____
_____

And third, we have Nancy. Straight yet relaxed shoulders complement Nancy's pleasant smile. Her head and neck are erect, allowing her eyes to glance freely around the room. Nancy's outfit is always in good taste, and she is well groomed.

Your impression is:

_____
_____
_____
_____
_____

Okay, now let's compare our answers!

Susy, bless her heart, appears to be slouchy. Her posture tells you that she has a poor self-image and lacks confidence. She tends to be shy, quiet, and keeps to herself. Her clothing tells you she wants to cover up and hide her real self from others. Susy has potential if she is willing to start liking who she is.

Angela is unmistakably on the road to arrogance. Her uplifted head and chest make her appear very self-confident, which she may or may not be. It could be a cover-up! Angela's prideful and cocky attitude is reflected in her carriage and her clothing. All of these combined make her unreachable, hardly the type you would expect to be true friends with.

Nancy has learned how to be herself. She likes who she is, knowing she has good characteristics and some not-so-good characteristics that she is working on. This is reflected in her confident posture and appearance. Nancy is a natural—friendly, approachable, and realistic.

Which impression do you want to give others through your posture? What does your body positioning tell others about you? Are you confident, insecure, or arrogant? Friendly, unapproachable, or withdrawn? Of the three examples we discussed, which one are you? I am a Nancy. Nancy's posture, appearance, and personality suit me best. I try to be friendly and kind to others. Most of all, like Nancy, I am confident in who I am. But I haven't always been. I learned to be. You can, too.

Your Confidence Affects Your Posture

Every one of us has reasons to stand up straight and feel confident about who we are. Can you think of some? How about these:

- You are special and unique—one-of-a-kind!
- You are a winner and can do all things.
- You are a woman—a prize creation of God.
- You are alive! You are a human life and every life has value.
- Perhaps you have achievements and accomplishments associated with your name—academics, sports, animals, arts, crafts, church or community work.
- As a Christian, you are a child of God and the Holy Spirit lives in you.
- Everyone has natural gifts and talents. God has put His gifts and talents inside of you to be used for Him.
- You are loved and accepted into the family of God!

I don't know you personally, but I am sure you have many reasons to feel confident. The Bible says in Proverbs 3:26 that the Lord is your confidence. He is the foundation and the purpose for your confidence. Your other achievements, talents, gifts, and relationships are just an added bonus. You can believe in the person God has made you by putting your confidence in Him. Knowing that God loves and accepts you is also a confidence builder!

In Hebrews 10:35 we are instructed not to throw away confidence in ourselves or confidence in God, because it has great rewards!

Now that we know how to develop confidence, let's show that confidence in our posture.

Six Points to Perfect Posture

1. Hold your head directly above your shoulders. Don't lean your neck forward or backward. Your chin should be parallel with the floor.

2. Pull your shoulders slightly back. This does not mean shoulders go upward to the ears! Back means *back*.

3. Lift your rib cage. Take a deep breath and feel your rib cage lift. Now hold it there, using the lower rib area to breathe. *Don't* take a deep breath

and hold it. Your ribs and lungs are not connected. You can lift your rib cage and breathe normally at the same time. Also, it is nearly impossible for your shoulders to slump forward if your rib cage is lifted properly.

4. Tuck your pelvic bone forward. If you have a tendency to stand with your backside sticking out, gently rotate your pelvis area forward. Again, don't exaggerate! This is a good time to tighten your abdominal muscles. This will give you a slender appearance.

5. Let your arms hang naturally at your sides. When you walk, swing your arms slightly. This should be a controlled movement. No floppy arms allowed! Your arm swing will naturally be in proportion to your step size. For example, when you are in a hurry and your step is larger, your arm swing increases just a bit. Small steps go with a small swing. The palms of your hands face the sides of your thighs. Practice this by slightly brushing your center finger against the sides of your legs as you walk. Fingers are relaxed, pointing downward rather than making a fist.

6. Now the icing on the cake: your facial expression! What is your face revealing to others? Take a good look. Even go so far as to practice pleasant expressions in front of the mirror. Happy smiling!

Body Alignment

From a side view, perfect body alignment looks like Figure 2-1.

If someone drew a line down the center of your body, would the line be this straight? The perfect lineup is head, ear, neck, shoulder, elbow, hip, knee, and ankle. Adjust your own body alignment where it is needed.

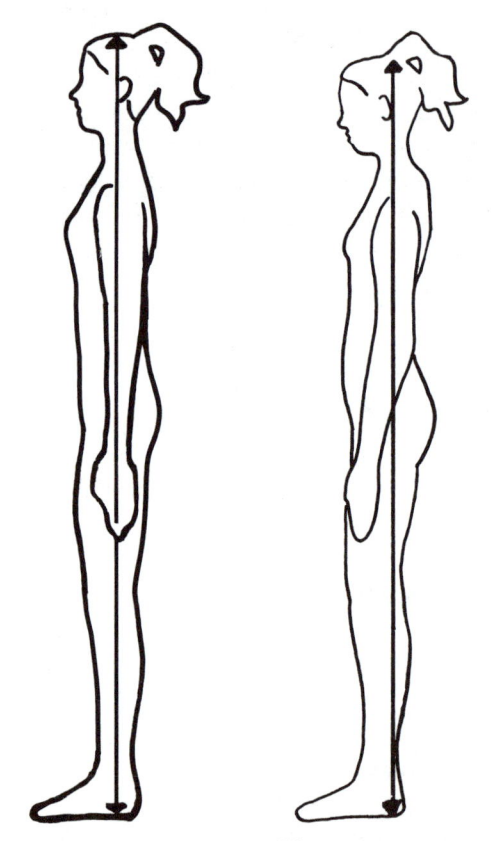

Figure 2-1. Correct Alignment

Figure 2-2. Incorrect Alignment

Here are the positive results of good posture:

- You appear confident and poised.
- You have more vocal power.
- Your inner organs have plenty of room to function.
- You will look slender and more professional with proper alignment.
- Your clothing will have a nicer fit.
- Proper posture can help relieve stress on your body.
- You will feel better about yourself.

Posture Exercises

If you are finding some of the posture points a challenge, try these exercises for quicker and better results. Like all the muscles in your body, your "posture muscles" need to be exercised in order to become toned. Do these exercises regularly!

1. *Shoulder blades.* Using both hands, take a heavy can or a three-pound dumbbell and lift it directly over your head. Bending your elbows, slowly lower the can behind your head, down toward the middle of your shoulder blades. Hold for thirty seconds, then slowly raise the can to the starting position. Repeat five to ten times.

2. *Lower back straightener.* The invisible chair sit! Lean your back against a wall with your feet shoulder width apart and twelve inches away from the baseboard. Slowly slide down the wall until you are in a sitting position. Press the small of your back against the wall. Hold as long as possible, then return to the starting position. Repeat five to ten times.

3. *Swayback.* Lean your back against a wall with your feet shoulder width apart and ten inches from the baseboard. Now bend all the way to the floor, keeping your hips against the wall and your knees slightly flexed. Slowly, one vertebra at a time, lift to an upright position, pressing each vertebra to the wall. Your head should be the last part of your body to touch the wall. Repeat five to ten times.

4. *Strengthening the back.* Lie with your back flat on the floor and with your hands above your head, your knees up and your feet flat on the floor. Now press your tummy down toward the floor so that the small of your back presses against the floor. Hold. Repeat ten times.

5. *Upper back and arm muscles.* Stand in your perfect-posture position. Lift your arms out to your sides, then move them backwards as far as you're able to reach. Hold fifteen seconds, then relax. Repeat the exercise ten times.

6. *Balance and posture.* Stand straight and tall, applying the "six points to perfect posture." Now slowly raise your right leg about twelve inches off the floor. Hold for a few seconds and lower your leg. Repeat with your left leg ten times. If you are feeling really brave, stand on one leg and hold the other one out in front of you, then in back of you. Happy balancing!

7. *Shoulders.* I have done this one many times, so I know it will help keep your shoulders back. Take a long piece of masking tape and attach one end to the front part of your left shoulder. Now pull your shoulders back into the correct position. Bring the masking tape back around the shoulder, all the way across your back, and attach the other end to the front of your right shoulder. Now every time you relax your shoulders and they want to slump forward, they will pull on the tape. What a great reminder! In case you're wondering—yes, you do attach the tape to your bare skin, and then put a shirt over it so the tape can't be seen. Try it out at home before you ever wear the tape in public!

Standing

You might be saying, "Now that I'm holding my body right, what do I do with my feet?" Great question. There are two ways to stand that will give you a poised and confident appearance. The key ingredient in both of these positions is this: Keep your knees and ankles close together!

1. *Side-by-side stance.* Put your feet together pointing straight forward with your knees touching, if possible, and slightly flexed, not locked. Your

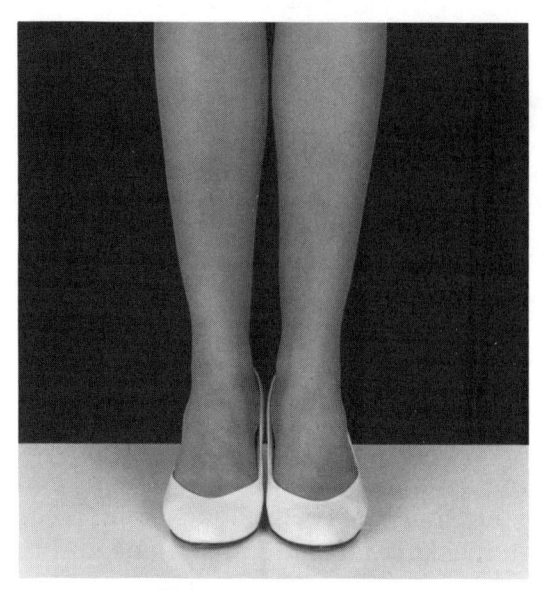

Side-by-Side Stance

weight should be equally balanced on both feet. Leaning on one leg looks a bit sloppy and unattentive.

2. *Model's stance.* In this stance, only your front foot faces directly forward, while your back foot is at a forty-five-degree angle. The heel of your front foot should be touching the arch of your back foot. Your weight should be on your back foot, allowing your front knee to be slightly flexed, not locked. This makes your knee appear more feminine. A slight turning of your hips, about a three-quarter angle, gives your hips a thinner appearance, and also gives a silhouette of your bust line. With your weight on the back foot, you will be free to take your first step with the front foot. That's how it is done in modeling!

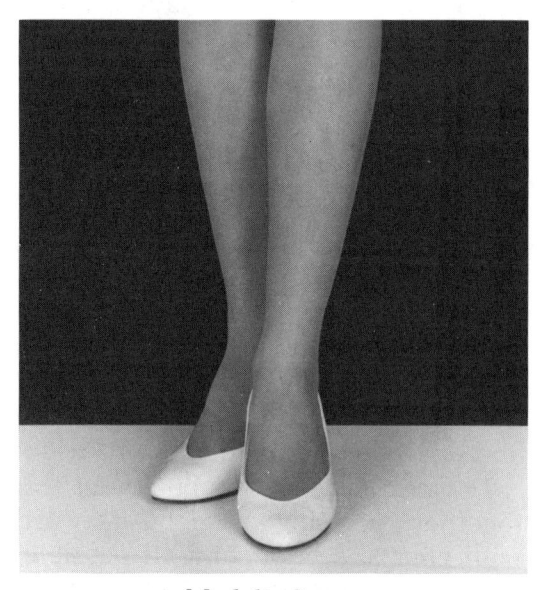

Now, where can you put these two stances to use? How about here:

- In front of a group.
- Waiting in a line (like the school lunch line or the theater).
- At a formal occasion.
- On a date.
- At an interview.
- When having your picture taken.
- When in a fashion show.
- Anytime!

Walking Right

I know, you learned to walk years ago. But I have a few hints to share that may improve the style of your walk. Everyone knows that as ladies we are to walk with one foot *directly* in front of the other. But do you know why? Try this simple test.

Stand with your feet about eight inches apart. Now draw an imaginary line across your hips, down one leg, across the feet, and up the other leg, back to where you started. What shape did you just create? Right! A rectangle. Now try this: Place your left foot directly in front of your right as if you were taking a step. Now draw another line across your hips, down one leg, to your feet, and up the other leg. What shape did you draw this time? A triangle or a V shape. Considering both shapes, which one is more feminine? I

Model's Stance

hope you said the V shape. When you walk with your feet placed one directly in front of the other, it is more feminine as well as more graceful because of the shape.

Toed-Out Toes

You may have noticed something about your feet. When you take a step, your foot is slightly "toed out." In other words, the position of your foot is at a slight angle. This is for balance and it is normal. If you were to walk a straight line, the inner edge of your heel and the inner edge of your big toe knuckle would be just touching the line. Notice the line is not running through the middle of the big toe. (*See* Figure 2-3.)

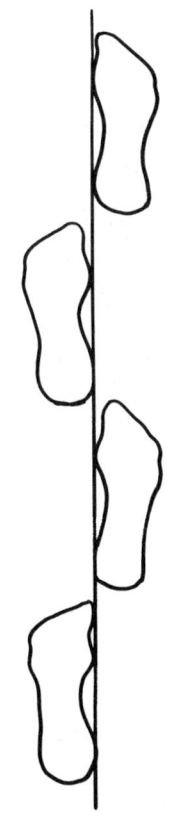

Figure 2-3. Walking with toes slightly turned out.

You will be better balanced if you keep your weight evenly distributed on both feet as you walk. Slightly flex your knees. Don't lock them with each step. You are after a smooth, gliding look to your walk, not a bounce.

Control Those Hips!

Your hip movement needs to be controlled. With your hip facing forward, bring each leg through the hip joint smoothly, making sure you don't throw your hip joint sideways with each step. Doing this will keep you from looking floppy, and will also make your clothes hang better.

Avoid leaning into your walk. Remember, keep your rib cage lifted and your chin parallel to the floor. Again, your arm swing should be natural, with your palms facing your outer thighs. The average length of one step is usually one and one-half times your foot length. Of course your step length will be altered depending upon the quickness of your steps.

One final tip on walking: Please don't drag your heels when you walk. This will detract from your walking style and wear the heels off your shoes very quickly.

Walk With the Lord

We have just talked about the kind of walking we do with our legs and feet. But have you ever heard anyone ask the question "How is your walk with the Lord?" Walk with the Lord? What does that mean? Here the term *walk* refers to a relationship. "How is your relationship with the Lord?" is what the person is really asking.

You are in a special relationship with

God, on a continuous journey through life with the One who loves you the most. This relationship, unlike others, will last forever. Jesus has promised that He will never leave you or turn away from you. The Lord is here to be your best friend. Are you spending time with Him daily, talking over every single problem facing you, sharing your joys and disappointments?

Just as we must do if we want to get to know a new friend at school better, we must spend time getting to know God. It is time well spent. Talk to Him. Read His Word. Your relationship or walk with the Lord is meant to be your best walk ever.

Turning Around

I have seen girls get their feet and legs twisted up and even trip over their own feet when they turn around. So, if you know *how* you are going to turn, it will be smooth sailing.

To do this turn you must plan ahead. Know where you are going to turn. This is called "spotting." In other words, find the spot where you are going to make the turn. Then, instead of taking a full-sized step, place the heel of one foot directly in front of the tip of the toes of your other foot. (*See* Figure 2-4.) There will be only an inch or so of space between your feet. Now lift up on the balls of your feet. Barely lifting your heels, turn halfway around so that you are facing the opposite direction. (*See* Figure 2-5.) If when you begin your turn your right foot is forward, then you will turn to your left. Likewise, if your left foot is forward you will turn to your right.

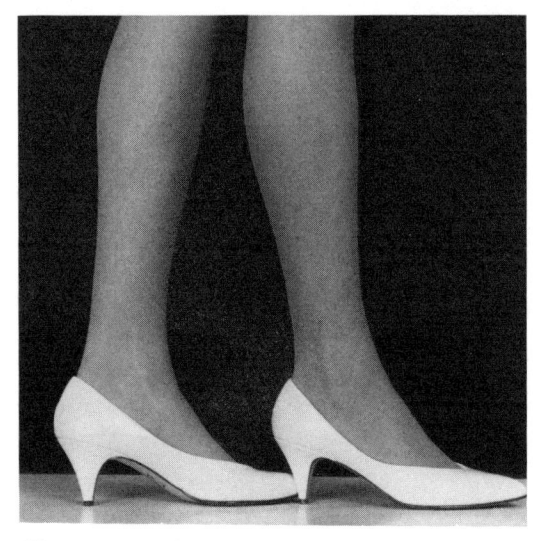

Figure 2-4. Preparing to turn, touch heel and toe.

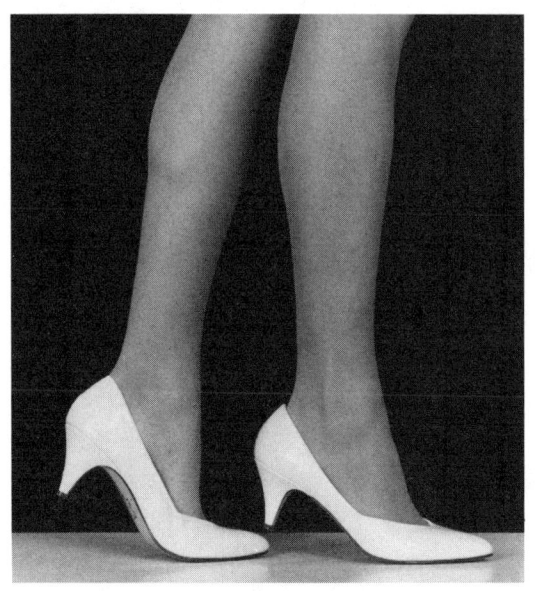

Figure 2-5. Lift up on the balls of your feet, slowly turning in the opposite direction of your front foot.

Did you notice that after you turned, your back foot was your front foot and your front foot was your back? Be sure your back foot ends up in a forty-five-degree angle, as it is in the model's stance. In fact, you should be in the model's stance when you end the turn. Remember: Practice makes perfect—or *close* to perfect, anyway!

Sitting Pretty

Sitting can be made much less clumsy by applying a few simple techniques. As you approach a chair, spot where you will be turning around in order to sit down. Go ahead and turn. Hopefully you will end up very close to the front edge of the chair. Now back up until you can feel your calf touching the edge of the chair. (*See* Figure 2-6.) You know the chair is there because you can feel it. Right? Now you don't have to look over your shoulder at the chair or turn to touch it to be sure it is behind you. We have all probably experienced the embarrassment of falling flat on our behinds because someone pulled a chair out from under us. Ouch! But when you are touching the chair with your calf, you can be sure you will have a safe landing.

Now using those power-packed thigh muscles, lower yourself slowly, and with much control, to the front part of the chair. Lower yourself straight down. Don't lean forward. Keep your back straight from the waist up. If you are sitting all the way to the back of the chair, then you went too far! Ideally, you want to be on the front third of the chair. (*See* Figure 2-7.) If you are wearing a dress, hold the sides of the skirted part forward before you sit down. Do this right where your hands hang to your sides. Don't tuck your dress under your buttocks—it will only draw attention where you don't want it!

Let's see, I left you sitting on the front of your chair. No, you don't have to stay that way! Place your palms,

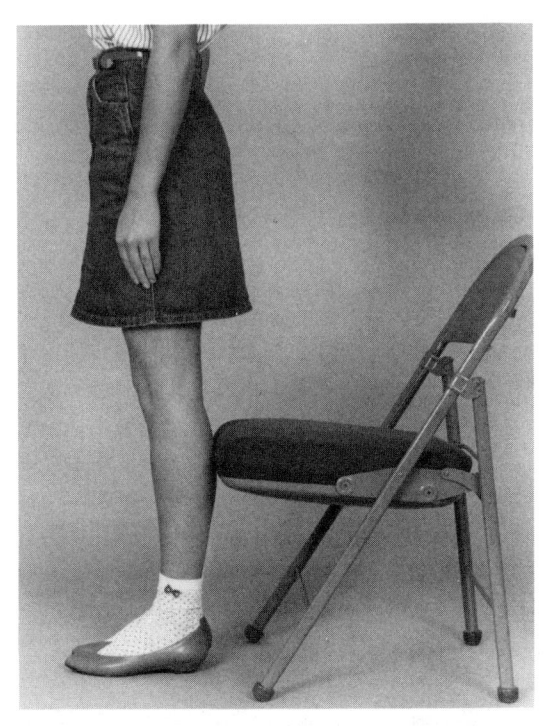

Figure 2-6. In preparing to sit down, touch your calf to the front edge of the chair.

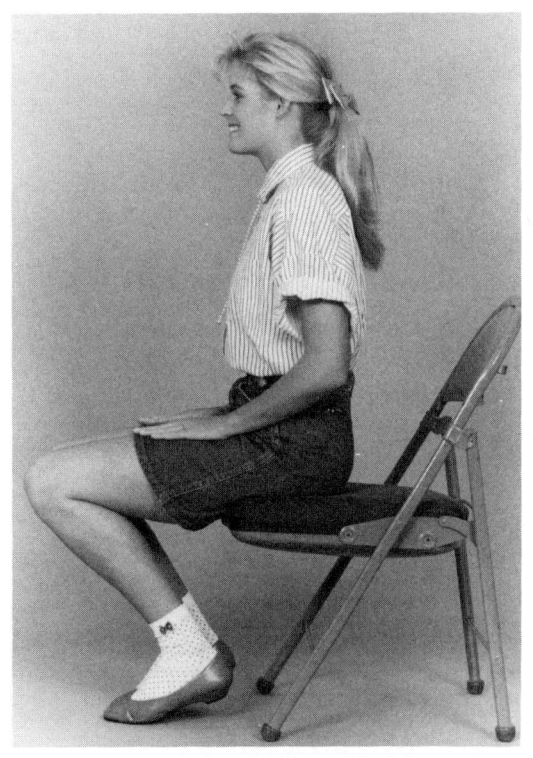

Figure 2-7. With your palms facedown on your thighs, lower yourself so you are sitting on the front one-third of the chair.

with your fingers closed, on the tops of your upper thighs. Gently lift your body, using your hands as resistance, and move to the back of the chair. Adjust yourself so you're comfortable. Now put your hands together and try one of these suggestions:

1. Place your hands together, one on top of the other, with both palms down. (*See* Figure 2-8.)
2. Place your hands together with the bottom palm up and the top palm down on top of the other hand.
3. Loosely interlock fingers from both hands, creating a V shape.
4. Avoid crossing your arms, playing with your hair, or fussing with your clothes.

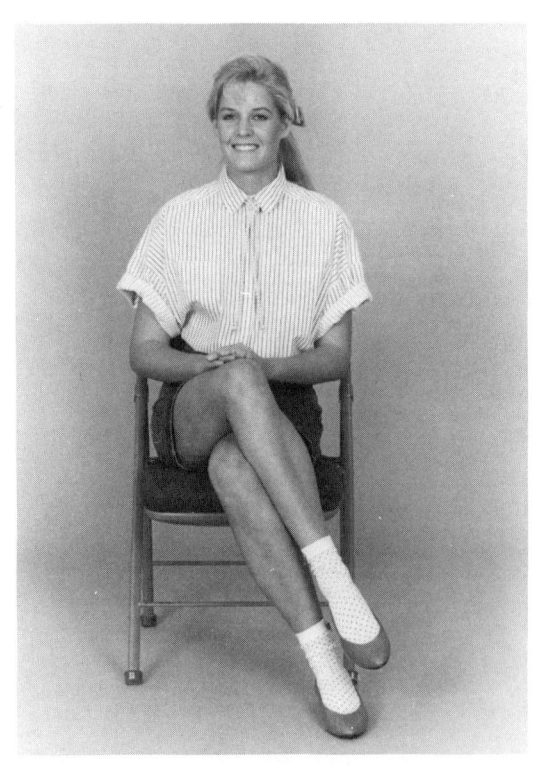

Figure 2-8. Kara is displaying a good sitting pose, keeping her hands one on top of the other, palms down, crossed legs close together, giving a slenderizing and polished appearance.

Now for your feet. Try any of these positions for a very together look:

1. Line up both feet directly under your knees, feet together.
2. Place both feet off to one side, ankles close together.
3. Cross your feet at the ankles. Be aware of keeping your knees from falling open. Position your feet off to one side.
4. Crossing your knees can be tough on the blood circulation in your legs. But since most of us cross our legs anyway, we can at least try this technique that eases up on the circulation. Cross your legs above your knees and try to lay your top leg on your bottom leg. This also gives a slenderizing look to your legs. (*See* Figure 2-8.)
5. Avoid twisting your feet around the leg of the chair.
6. Avoid sitting with one foot sideways on top of your other knee, the way most guys do!

When you are ready to get up out of the chair, uncross your legs and/or ankles, and place them directly beneath your knees. If they are too far under the chair you will have a hard time getting up. You might even want to try placing one foot a little bit ahead of the other. Place your palms on top of your thighs and use them as resistance to push yourself up. Try lifting with your back straight, rather than diving forward in order to get momentum to lift out of the chair. These sitting secrets may take an extra bit of practice, but you will be glad you took the time to perfect them.

Managing Stairs

Just a word on going up and down stairs. Using your correct posture, try to glide, rather than bounce, up and down the steps. You do this by not locking your knees every time you take a step. Locking your knees causes a jerk in your movement. Keep your knees slightly bent. To help you get the feel of not locking your knees with each step, practice walking around the room with both of your knees bent. Feel the control in your thighs? That's where true control for a smooth glide up or down the stairs really is—in your thighs.

When you are moving up the stairs, your heel touches the step first and then your toe touches the step. Use your toes to lift you up to the next step. Reach with your toes to the lower step when moving down the stairs. Be sure you place your entire foot on the step.

You may want to try walking on the stairs at an angle. This is not as difficult as it may sound. Keep your upper body fairly straight forward, while you turn your lower body at a slight angle. It doesn't matter whether you turn to the right or the left. Concentrate on looking downward at the steps with your eyes only, not with your entire head. Walking the stairs at an angle adds a touch of dignity and style to your appearance.

Visual Graces— Looking Good!

A beautiful part of being a woman is knowing how to make the most of what you have been blessed with. Each of us has a special purpose, and each of us is unique. The visual grace suggestions that follow will help you as you strive to be your very best. They will also help you to look your best in social situations so that you can feel comfortable in the way you handle yourself.

1. Be aware of others around you and how your actions might affect them. Allow others to go first. Let them know they count! Be generous with kind acts and good deeds. Let your love for the Lord show through your actions.

2. Carry your handbag with grace. Avoid a "slung over the shoulder" look. If the purse has a long handle, allow it to hang under your arm; if it has short handles, carry it by the handles. Use leather or heavy-material handbags in the winter and lighter-material bags in the summer. As for color, choose lighter shades in the spring and summer, darker shades in the colder months.

3. When carrying a clutch bag, keep your index finger along the top of the bag, pointing your finger to the floor. This gives your hand and arm a long, graceful look. Naturally it will be hard to do this if your clutch bag is stuffed with all the goodies you just can't do without. Perhaps you could try a larger purse!

4. When reaching for an object, rather than leading with your fingertips, bend your hand at the wrist and lead with your wrist. When nearing the object you are about to pick up or touch, gracefully straighten your wrist, using your thumb and middle fingers to pick up the object. If you must bend to pick something up, bend at your knees rather than at your waist. When you bend at your waist you may put pressure on your lower back and unavoidably make your bottom stick out. So, go for the knees!

5. It is much more feminine to cover your mouth with the back of your hand when you yawn, though using the front of your hand is all right. Cup your hand, keeping your fingers

straight and closed together. Always say, "Excuse me." Keep your elbow to your side and your fingers at a pretty angle.

6. When entering a room you are unfamiliar with, pause in your model's stance. Look around the room with a pleasant expression on your face. (Remember, first impressions happen only once.) Then, when you decide where you want to sit, walk confidently there. Avoid table hopping and seat switching! Look confident, not confused.

7. When putting on your coat, do it in a graceful and ladylike manner. Don't swing your coat over the top of your head! Hold the center of the collar in your right hand, gliding your left arm into the left-arm sleeve. Then place your left hand on the left lapel and drop your coat downward. Your left hand will now be up near the top of your shoulder. The armhole for the right sleeve should be in a good position to easily put your right arm into the right coat sleeve! Bring the right shoulder of the coat up as you put the coat on, and adjust the fit. Start to button the coat at the top and button downward. I hope you don't get your left and right confused. You might end up with your coat on backwards!

When removing your coat, unbutton from the bottom up. Then place your hands on the lapels of the coat and lift it over your shoulders. Drop your arms behind your back and tug slightly at the cuffs if the coat won't slide off. Tug behind you, not in front. When the coat is off, fold, hang up, or place it on the back of your chair. Please don't toss your coat in a convenient corner! You may be wondering, if you are with a guy, should he help you with your coat? Absolutely! In fact, assume that he will help you, even if you must politely ask him to.

8. Shake hands with a firm grasp, not a limp hand. This tells the other person that you are confident and also pleased to meet him or her. Yes, even females shake hands! If you are seated, standing to be introduced to someone is optional. It used to be that ladies remained seated and men stood when being introduced to someone. However, standing is an honorable gesture for a male or female. The choice is yours.

9. Put your makeup on in private, not in public. This even includes lip gloss and combing your hair! Show others the "finished" product, the "put together" you. Always prepare yourself at home or in the privacy of a rest room. This may be hard for those of you girls at school who think you always have to use your brushes before each class period ends.

10. When people speak to you, look into their eyes. I know this won't be hard if it is a cute guy you are talking to! Blinking your eyes shows attention, interest, and adds sparkle to your eyes. Listen to others' opinions, and accept people with a warm heart.

11. Plan ahead! When a guy opens a door for you, be in the right position to avoid embarrassing both of you. Having to duck under his arm or walk around to the other side of him in order to go through the door should let you know you were in the wrong place. When you are approaching a door, think which side of him you need to be on in order to simply stroll through the opened door. Get on that side! It would be wonderful if the guy knew about door opening also, but if not, you be the one to make it flow

smoothly. And don't forget to say thank you!

12. Snapping and chomping on a piece of gum doesn't look too great. Dispose of your gum properly. Use a waste can or wrap your gum in a piece of paper and put it in your purse. Avoid the temptation to stick it somewhere.

13. Being fun and being obnoxious are two different things. Watch your manners. There is a time to kick back and a time to act respectfully.

14. When opening or closing a door, reach for the knob by leading with your wrist; control the turning of the knob for less noise. Gently close the door, keeping your hand on the knob.

15. Show respect and patience for those who are serving you, such as teachers, waitresses, salespersons, janitors, cafeteria workers, secretaries, operators, and so on. Be kind, helpful, and understanding as if *you* were serving *them*. Say please, thank you, and excuse me when appropriate. You will feel good by making them feel good.

Inner Visual Poise

By now you have a great start on becoming a beautifully poised young lady. And that is wonderful—for the outside. But have you ever thought about what it means to be poised on the inside?

We defined *visual poise* as "the outward control of your body movements." How do you think we can define *inner visual poise*?

When I think of the women I have known who are poised inwardly, the word that comes to my mind is *gracious*. A gracious woman is one who is very thankful for all she has. She is rarely greedy or jealous over the belongings of others. She is content. She has a quiet and gentle spirit about her. She is a good listener and doesn't get angry very easily. She is kind, courteous, graceful, and she does things in good taste. She is merciful and shows compassion to others. Not only does she have outward control, she also has inward control.

Are you on your way to becoming a gracious woman? Sure, it won't happen overnight, but it's not impossible! When you are practicing your outer visual poise techniques, don't forget to practice your inner visual poise. A gracious woman is precious in the sight of God and others.

BEAUTIFULLY CREATED

VISUAL POISE

Project Page

1. There is no such thing as a wrong body type. We are all graceful in different situations. Name someone you know who is graceful in these situations:

   baseball_____
   track_____
   volleyball_____
   ballet_____
   bowling_____
   personal mannerisms_____
   walking_____

2. In what areas could you improve your visual poise? How would this give you more self-confidence?_____
   _____
   _____
   _____
   _____

3. Posture gives off messages. Describe someone you know who is a Susy, an Angela, and a Nancy. Which are you? What messages does your posture give about you?_____
   _____
   _____
   _____
   _____
   _____
   _____

4. Secure a string or tape measure down the center of a full-length mirror. Stand sideways. Check to see how your posture lines up!

5. Write yourself a reminder to stand and sit up straight. Put the note in a schoolbook or tape it to the inside of your locker at school.

6. Try each posture exercise daily for a month. Notice the improvement?

VISUAL POISE

7. Draw a chalk line on the sidewalk or stretch a string across the floor for a distance of about thirty feet. Put a chair at one end of the string. Now practice walking with one foot directly in front of the other all the way to the chair, do a heel-toe turn, sit in the chair correctly, then stand and walk back to your original starting point. Putting these moves together and getting them down will help make them a habit.

8. Practice applying each of the "visual graces." Can you think of others to add to this list?_____
   _____
   _____

9. Describe what it means to be gracious. Do you know someone who is gracious? What do you admire about her?
   _____
   _____
   _____
   _____

10. How would you describe your "walk with the Lord"?
    _____an effortless slow walk   _____a brisk walk
    _____a slow jog   _____a fast run

11. List two ways you could improve your pace._____
    _____
    _____

3 SENSATIONAL SKIN
Sensible Steps to Great-Looking Skin

Skin. Just another miracle given to you from the Lord, the Great Designer. Ever think of your skin that way? A miracle? Well, it's true. Your skin does so much more than just sit there on your bones and hold your insides together!

Do you know what the largest living organ of your body is? Right—your skin. That was easy. But do you know all of the important functions this organ performs? To begin with, your skin is the largest waste organ of your body. It perspires, cleansing your body of harmful poisons and toxins. But at the same time it holds in natural body fluids you need for that healthy look!

While your skin is regulating fluids, it is also regulating your body temperature, keeping it, on the average, at 98.6 degrees. Producing vitamin D and certain hormones is also the skin's job.

Your skin contains blood vessels that cause your face to redden when you blush. It also has sweat glands, hair follicles, oil glands, and tough, highly elastic fibers that help keep it young looking. Your skin serves as a shield against germs and pollutants.

If you could peel it all off, your skin would weigh about six pounds. It varies in thickness. Can you guess where it is thickest? Your palms and the soles of your feet. Where is it thinnest? Under your eyes, on your eyelids, and the front of your neck. Did you guess right?

Perhaps the most life-enriching characteristic of your skin is its sensitivity to touch. Skin picks up messages from others and from your environment, and sends them on to your brain. A slap, a pinprick, a loving stroke, or a teddy bear hug—the skin knows them all. I think everyone's skin likes hugs the best. Did you know that we all need at least four hugs a day? Hugs keep us healthy. Be sure you give away plenty each day!

Your skin has two layers. The outer layer is called the *epidermis*. The inner layer is called the *dermis*. Both layers are unique, yet they are closely interlaced to do their jobs together. The outer layer is surfaced with tiny oil-releasing openings called *pores*. This layer serves as a protective covering for the sensitive inner layer. In exchange, the inner layer feeds, moisturizes, and supplies blood to the outer layer. Sounds like they use the buddy system!

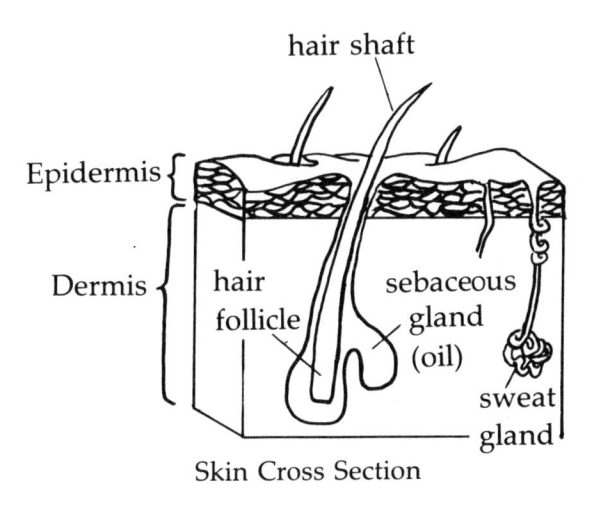

Since this miracle organ called skin is so important, you need to give it lots of attention and lots of care. Skin is completely dependent upon the person wearing it. That's you! You want your skin—and not just the part everyone sees all the time—to look its best for as long as you have it . . . but it can't do it by itself. It needs you. Your teen years are the perfect time to begin caring for your skin.

Skin Types

Your first step on the road to good-looking skin is to identify your type of skin. This will tell you what specific care it needs. Do you know your skin type? Look at your facial skin. Can you pinpoint which of the following fits you?

Oily Skin. This skin type produces an excess of oil, causing the pores to be larger to accommodate the constant flow of oil from the sebaceous glands in the dermis. Oily skin usually shines; it tends to form blackheads and whiteheads and to break out easily. This, of course, is because of the high amount of oil in the skin. Oily skin is a bit thicker than the other skin types and has a coarser texture. The big plus is that it is less prone to wrinkles in later years.

Normal Skin. This skin type manages to maintain a good balance of natural moisture and a moderate flow of oil. Therefore, its pores are medium sized and it seldom breaks out.

Dry Skin. Because it produces even less oil, dry skin has small pores, flakes easily, and shows wrinkles sooner. It tends to be thin and finely textured, so dry skin needs extra moisture. It also needs extra protection from the sun.

Combination Skin. This is the most common skin type and often combines all three of the previous types. It is usually oily across the forehead and down the center of the face. This is called the T zone. The other areas of the face may be normal or dry. The combinations vary.

Skin Type Test

If you are still unsure about your skin type, or you just can't seem to identify which description fits you best, try this simple test.

Thoroughly cleanse your face right before you go to bed. (*See* "Skin Care: The Basics" for complete instructions.) Use a mild astringent or freshener. Do not use a moisturizer. In the morning when you first wake up, lay a tissue over your entire face. Now press the tissue against your skin at your forehead, cheek, sides of your nostrils, upper lip, and chin. Hold it at each spot for three to four seconds. Now lift the tissue and hold it up to the light. Where is it oily? Where is it dry? A slight bit of oil is normal; no oil on the tissue indicates dry skin; a significant amount of oil means you have oily skin. Now can you pinpoint your skin type? Hopefully so.

Nourishing Your Skin

Since it is a living organ, your skin needs to be fed. We all know how to feed our hungry stomachs, but how do we feed our skin?

Ideal conditions, both internal and external, nourish our skin, giving it a healthier appearance. External conditions, such as climate, feed our skin. Humid climates leave your skin less dry. Climates where the sun's rays are less penetrating will result in fewer wrinkles.

Internal conditions, such as eating all the right foods and drinking lots of water, will also feed your skin what it hungers for.

But, since we don't all live in the ideal skin climate, or eat the way we should, and drink soda instead of water, we need to look elsewhere for a little help in skin nutrition. This is where skin-care products come in. Proper skin-care products make a great meal for your skin.

Choose skin-care products that suit your type of skin so that they will be effective. For example, oily skin will need products that are oil free, whereas dry skin will need products that contain extra moisture. The products are usually marked as to which skin type they are specifically designed for.

How do you decide which brand of skin-care products to use? It is easy to be swayed by pretty packaging. Plus, each company claims that theirs is the best. Ever feel confused? It is true that there are many good skin-care lines on the market. I highly recommend selecting a product that is allergy tested and 100 percent fragrance free. Allergy tested means the product has been stripped of all ingredients that might irritate even the most sensitive skin. Fragrance free, of course, means that no fragrance has been added. This keeps the product pure and eliminates the possibility of a negative reaction with your skin.

I also recommend that you use products that are from the same company. When I first begin working with individual girls, I ask them what skin-care products they are using and, almost every time, they tell me they use a little of this brand, a little of that, a little of still another brand. You won't get maximum results if you use a mixture of skin-care brands. (I'm talking about skin-care products and foundation, not makeup.) Cosmetic companies have designed their products to be used together in order to benefit your skin.

Shop around before you buy. Asking

questions of a salesperson does not obligate you to buy the products. When you decide, buy the smallest quantities possible if you've never used them before. Then give them time to work. Many companies suggest using their line for at least three weeks. By then you will either see an improvement or get an undesirable reaction. If you react negatively to a product, stop using it right away.

As I will discuss in the next chapter, it is not necessary to spend lots of money on your makeup—blush, eye shadow, lip gloss. It is important, however, that you use a high-quality skin-care line, even if it means spending a few extra dollars. This is not to say that the most expensive products are necessarily the best. Read the labels and compare ingredients!

Skin Care: The Basics

Keeping your skin clear and healthy is a twice-a-day task—in the morning and at bedtime. But it's worth it. Get into the habit. Pull your hair away from your face, and let's get started!

1. *Cleansing.* Surface cleansing does just that—it cleanses the surface of your skin. Its main job is to remove old makeup, oils, dirt, and particles from the air that have collected on your skin. For this we use a commercial product. Cleansers come in bars, lotions, or creams. Some are rinsed off with water, some are tissued off. You will have to decide which you like best and which your skin responds to the best. Try to avoid using a cleanser that has a heavy oil base. Oil clogs your pores.

Water-based cleansing products are the best. How can you tell the difference? Simply read the list of ingredients on the package. If mineral oil or lanolin is listed as one of the first ingredients, find another cleanser. Baby oil and petroleum jellies are pure forms of oil. You should never use any straight-oil products on your face as cleansers or to remove eye makeup. Oil is not water soluble, and therefore does not dissolve. Many women have had severe eye problems when they used oil to remove eye makeup. The oil collects in the back of the eye area.

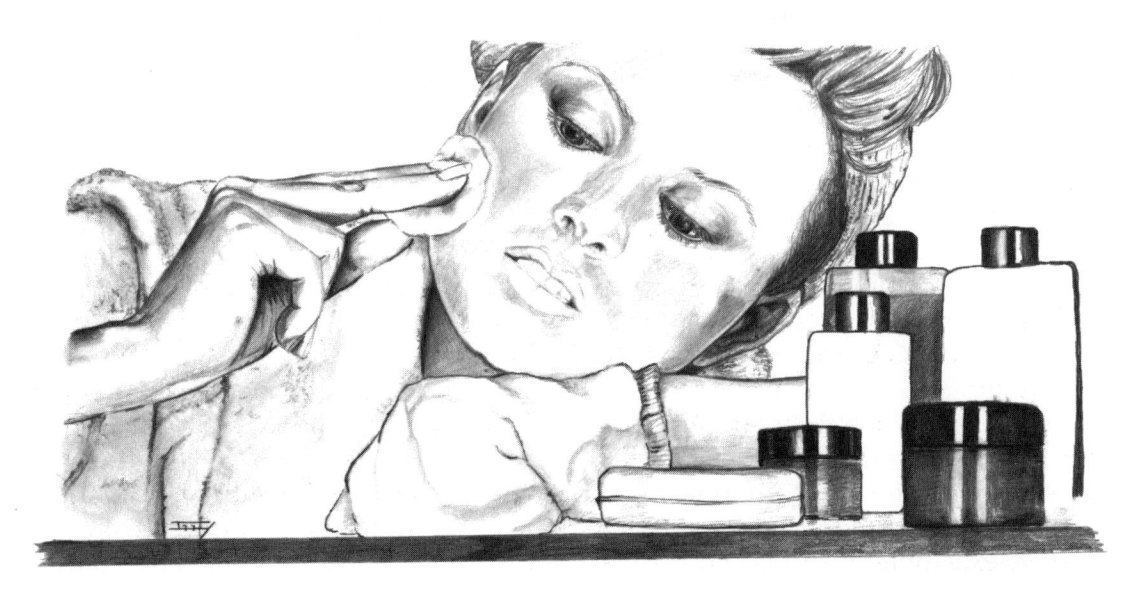

Eye-makeup removers must be non-oily or water based. When wearing makeup, use eye-makeup remover before your regular cleanser. This keeps mascara from being rubbed into your skin around your eye when you remove the rest of your makeup.

Your cleanser should leave your face feeling clean, not greasy. Because they are oil or grease based, many lotions and cold creams leave a residue on your skin's surface. That is hardly an effective cleanser, since it is supposed to be taking that stuff off your face.

Soaps are good surface cleansers but usually dry the skin because of the detergent in them. Nondetergent soaps are best for your facial skin—again, *read the labels*. Most quality companies make bar soap cleansers with no detergent, no fragrance, and no deodorant in them. These types of cleansers are a good choice. Do keep your facial cleansing bar and your hand soap separate.

Please note that cleansers and moisturizers are not the same thing. If a product claims to moisturize as well as clean, beware. A good cleanser will not leave residue on the surface of your skin. Besides, moisturizing is the third step, not part of the first.

Deep pore cleansers, made by only a few product lines, reach down into the inner layer of the skin and unclog pores by dissolving built-up oil, bacteria, and sweat residue. Deep pore cleanser should only be used after the surface cleanser. Certain facial masks act as deep pore cleansers. Details coming up.

If your skin tends to break out, you may use medicated cleansers. Ask your dermatologist or a good pharmacist to help you select the best one for you.

Now, exactly how should you use a cleanser? Using circular motions, gently work the cleanser into your skin. Never pull your skin or press on it hard. Facial skin and muscle tissue are very delicate and must be handled with TLC—tender loving care. (*See* Directional Chart, page 54.) Use your fingertips, or a washcloth. Makeup-remover pads are really not necessary. Be sure you are cleansing all the way to your hairline and under your chin.

Rinse the cleanser off thoroughly with lukewarm water. Hot water dries your skin and may overactivate your oil glands. After rinsing with warm water, slowly adjust the water temperature, making it cooler, not cold. Cold water may burst tiny blood vessels due to the shock of the temperature. Avoid extremes in temperature. Pat your face dry with a clean hand towel. Don't rub! And *never* go to bed with your makeup on.

2. *Astringent.* An astringent is an alcohol-based liquid that removes any cleanser still on your skin. It temporarily shrinks your pores and acts as a chemical exfoliator. Sounds technical, huh? *Exfoliate* means that the astringent removes the layer of dead skin cells that might have built up on the surface of your skin. These dead cells—meaning they no longer contain fluid—must be removed to allow the oil in your skin to flow properly to the top of the oil duct and out the pore.

Astringents are available in varying strengths to meet the needs of different skin types. Again, most product bottles are labeled according to the skin type they have been designed for. An astringent with a high level of alcohol would rob the natural moisture which dry skin needs but would balance out the overproduction of oil in oily skin. If your skin is normal or combination type, you need a medium-strength astringent. When you apply this product to your combination-type skin, use it only where your skin is oily, not where it is dry.

Dry skin does not need an alcohol-based product but a water-based product known as a freshener or toner. Fresheners and toners contain little or no alcohol. You can also use these on normal and combination skin if you find that an astringent is too harsh. Never, under any circumstances, use straight alcohol! Alcohol is much too strong in its natural form and can damage your skin.

Apply your astringent with a 100 percent cotton ball or pad. Other cosmetic puffs and pads contain tiny wood fibers because they are paper instead of cotton. The paper products can scratch your skin's sensitive surface.

To help dry breakout spots throughout the day, many cosmetic companies make astringent-filled tubes with applicator tips. These are handy for carrying in your purse or schoolbag. Thin absorbent tissues are also available in carry-along-size packets for blotting excess oil during the day. These are especially helpful if your skin is oily.

A special benefit of an astringent or freshener is that by clearing away excess cleanser and dead skin cells, it allows the moisturizer to be absorbed deep into your skin more effectively. This brings us to step three.

3. *Moisturizer*. The purpose of a moisturizer is to (1) seal in your skin's natural moisture, (2) soften your skin, and (3) replace lost moisture. There are many things that rob natural fluids from your skin: sun, wind, rain, perspiration, water, pollution, and of course, certain soaps. A moisturizer, then, helps to slow down the evaporation process of your skin's natural moisture and serves as a shield between the environment and the top layer of skin.

Do all skin types need moisture? Yes, they do—but the amount varies. Moisturizer comes in different weights. Oily skin needs only a lightweight, oil-free moisturizer. Normal skin requires medium-weight moisturizer, and dry skin responds best to a heavier moisturizer. Combination skin needs more than one weight.

Again, try not to use a moisturizer that has an oil base. Use a product that does not list oil as one of its primary ingredients. Moisturizer should not clog your pores but should give your skin a drink!

Since the area under your eyes and the skin on your neck have fewer oil glands, you should use special products in these two areas to provide extra moisture. There are many good eye and throat creams on the market.

Another area that loves special attention is your lips. Don't forget your lips! A lip balm or a touch of petroleum jelly (it's okay here) does a great job to soften and heal chapped lips—or to prevent chapping.

In addition to the benefits I've mentioned, moisturizer has a few extra features you should know about. Since it's the first product that soaks into your skin, moisturizer protects your skin's inner layers from potentially irritating dyes and chemicals in foundation.

This is a good place to talk about tinted moisturizers. I realize they sound like a wonderful idea, and they make skin care easier by combining the moisturizer and foundation color together, but for the reason I just mentioned, they need to be avoided. Foundation dyes and chemicals may irritate some skins. Allow your moisturizer to be absorbed into your skin on its own. Don't ever apply foundation without first applying your moisturizer!

Another benefit of moisturizer is that it makes way for smoother application of foundation.

So, there are the three steps to be used by all skin types: cleanser, astringent, and moisturizer.

Skin Care: The Specifics

Along with the basic daily care, there are a few special treatments to include on a weekly basis to help keep your skin clear and fresh. These simple techniques are not only effective, they are fun, too. A little extra care can make you feel your loveliest.

Facial Steaming

There are several methods for steaming your facial skin. The easiest method is to fill your bathroom sink three-quarters full of very hot water. Bend over the basin until your face is two to three inches above the water. Cover your head and the sink area with a bath towel to contain the steam. Slowly blow into the water to create more steam. The heat from the steam will cause your facial pores to open. This allows you to accomplish the main purpose of steaming—to flush out the pores.

Then, after two or three minutes, using lukewarm water, briskly splash your face over and over. When your pores are thoroughly flushed, slowly change the water temperature to cool in order to close the pores, returning them to normal. Once again, avoid extremes in water temperature.

If you can't get into the bathroom, heat water in a microwave or over the stove. Place the steaming water on the counter and tent a bath towel over your head. Then follow the instructions already given.

Another convenient way to get your pores open is to use a washcloth rinsed in very hot water. Lay the wrung-out cloth loosely on your face, gently pressing the cloth around your nose area. Repeat this process several times.

Automatic facial steamers or the use of a sauna are fun, but they can be inconvenient and costly. The other methods work just as well.

Facial Scrub

New skin cells are constantly being produced in the lower layers of the skin. As the plump new cells get closer to the skin's surface, they flatten out in shape. The flattened cells no longer contain liquid and are considered dead.

Removing this dead layer of skin allows the natural flow of oil to be released on the surface of the skin. Also, if these cells are not properly removed or sloughed off, they can give the skin a dull, ruddy appearance.

The process of removing dead skin cells is called *exfoliation*. As I mentioned earlier, an astringent helps to exfoliate by removing dead skin cells. To be sure the cells are completely removed, use a facial scrub. I call them scrubbies. Facial scrub is a cream-based product that contains tiny round particles. Don't use one that contains ground fruit pits or other rough ingredients. Your skin is very delicate and must be treated with care.

Use a scrub about once a week. I

recommend using it at night after cleansing your face. Simply wet your skin, then gently apply a penny-size dot of scrub to your entire face in a circular motion. (*See* Directional Chart, page 54.) Rinse thoroughly with warm water and follow with a mild astringent or freshener. Finish with a touch of moisturizer.

Dead skin cells do tend to shed naturally. Removing the cells with a facial scrub speeds the process, leaving the skin with a glowing, even appearance. If you are in the prepuberty or early puberty stage, using a washcloth when you cleanse will do the trick in removing unwanted skin cells. As your skin matures, add a facial scrub to your weekly routine. Everyone's body "time clock" is a bit different, so our skin needs will vary. Adjust your skin-care products and routine accordingly.

Facial Masks

There are several reasons we females dare to look totally ridiculous with funny-colored clay or peel-off gel glopped on our faces! Could this possibly lead to a more beautiful you? It is hard to imagine, but masks can be truly beneficial.

Not all masks serve the same purpose. Some cleanse, others slough off dead skin cells, moisturize, or even tone the skin. But all of them will leave your skin feeling soft and refreshed.

Choose a mask meant for your skin type and designed for the specific purpose you want to achieve. Read the labels carefully.

As a general rule, a mask will do the following:

- help firm the skin with its tightening effect
- stimulate the blood circulation which nourishes the skin cells and promotes healthy growth
- vacuum the pores and deep cleanse the skin, which helps to draw impurities to the surface
- moisturize dry skin or dry up oily skin, depending on the ingredients
- remove the top layer of dead skin cells

The instructions given with each commercial facial mask will tell you how and when to use it for the best results. Never apply a mask until your skin is thoroughly cleansed. Apply it *around* your eyes and lips, not on them! (*See* Figure 3-1.) Hold a damp, warm

Figure 3-1. Facial Mask

washcloth on your face to prepare your skin for the mask. Most masks need to be followed up with a moisturizer. Do not apply makeup for several hours.

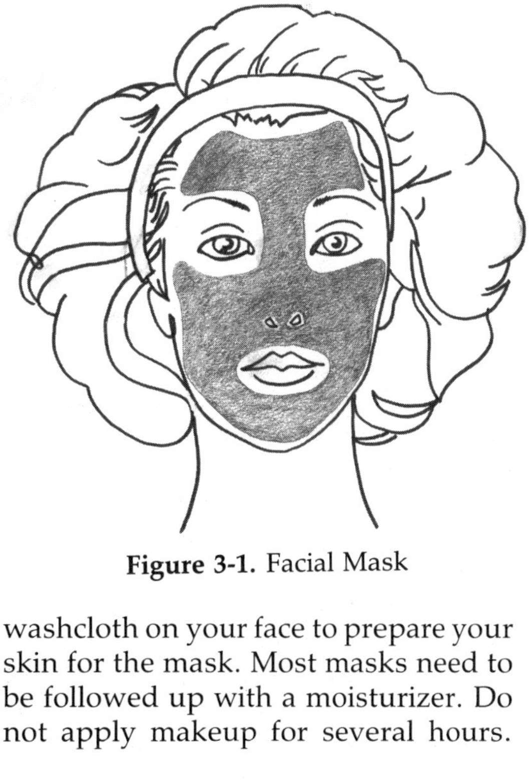

Homemade Masks

Besides the many masks available at your local drug or department store, here are three masks you can make at home.

Egg White Mask. Beat one egg white until it is stiff. Add one drop of lemon juice for a tingling feeling. Apply generously. Remove with warm water after the egg has tightened on your skin (about eight to ten minutes).

Oatmeal Mask. Put one cup of oatmeal into a blender. Blend at high speed to make the oats into a powder. Mix the powder with a little water to make a paste. Then apply it to your face. When the oatmeal no longer feels cool—about ten minutes—rinse it off. Store remaining oatmeal in an airtight bowl.

Yogurt Mask. Apply a thin layer of well-mixed, plain yogurt to your face. After ten minutes, rinse with warm water. Ah, what a feeling!

Looking at yourself in the mirror with a mask on might make you think of those silly things people wear to costume parties. There are all kinds of masks people use to disguise themselves. You know, masks are just that: false faces we use to hide behind to disguise our real selves.

We all wear masks of one kind or another. Maybe we're fearful but act tough. Maybe we're hurting but act happy, trying to look in control and totally cool.

Warning: Wearing these kinds of masks can be harmful. They stop you from being honest with yourself, others, and maybe even with God. Wearing masks in front of God is silly. God can see through every false image and disguise you might put on. The Lord knows the real you that hides behind the imitation face you wear.

I believe the Lord wants us to put away our masks in our relationship with Him and others. Jesus loves and accepts us just the way we are—but that doesn't mean there isn't room for improvement! But there's no need to try and fool Him. In our personal relationship with Jesus we can be ourselves, knowing with confidence that we will still be loved. Then we can use this confidence to remove our masks in our relationships with others. Gently washing away *these* kinds of masks will not only be good for your appearance but for your heart as well!

Directional Chart

When you are applying products to your face at any time, whether cleanser, exfoliating scrub, moisturizer, foundation, or a mask, you need to avoid pulling downward on your facial

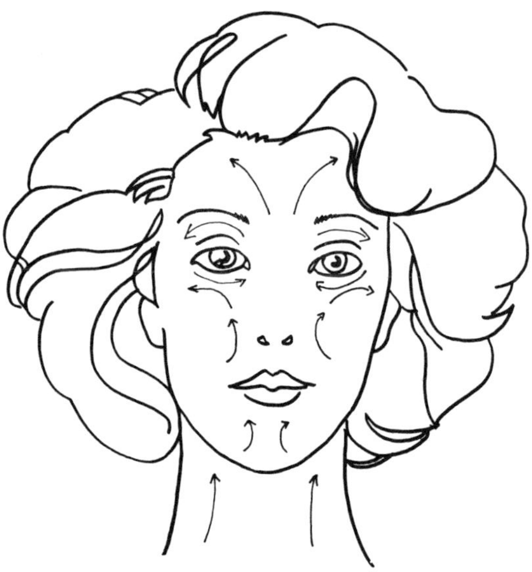

Figure 3-2. Directional Chart

skin. The following technique takes practice and concentration, but you can do it! Work in an upward and outward direction, using a circular motion. Since gravity pulls downward on your face, you need to work upward. The arrows on the diagram show the direction. They are:

- Chin: Circular motion moving upward.
- Cheeks: Upward motion, then outward toward the hairline.
- Forehead: Up and out toward the hairline.
- Eyes: On the eyelids, work from the tear duct area to the outer corner of the eye. Then under the eye, work from the outer corner back in toward the nose.
- Neck: Always work upward toward the jaw area.

Breakout

Pimples, blackheads, whiteheads—the skin's most unwanted visitors. Almost every face is affected by these annoying intruders.

Breakout is certainly no picnic. With each little bump, we feel more self-conscious and more like Cinderella *before* she gets the glass slipper! Not exactly a booster for a girl's self-image. At least most of us are in the same boat.

There are many things that affect our skin and promote breakout. Improper cleansing, heredity, skin type, emotions, too many fries and colas, and of course our menstrual cycles, just to name a few. Some we can control, some we cannot.

When it comes to a complexion complication, our best bet is to *clear it up* rather than *cover it up*. Running to the drugstore to buy those thick cover creams is not the answer! Carefully using the skin-care techniques we have already talked about; eliminating greasy foods, sugar, and caffeine; drinking six to eight glasses of water daily; taking a high-potency multiple vitamin daily; keeping our hands away from our faces; and getting plenty of rest are sure to bring better results.

Without getting too technical, following is a brief description of skin problems we all deal with, so you will understand what is happening.

Blackhead. When excess oil is produced, it causes the pore to get larger and the oil hardens, turns dark, and clogs the pore opening. Blackheads are best removed when you are steaming your facial skin, because the pores are open. Cover your fingertips with a tissue to prevent spreading bacteria, then gently press down on the area *around* the pore to force the hardened oil out. Do not squeeze. You can also use a blackhead extractor, a silver instrument with a small donut-looking tip that fits around the blackhead. Finish with repeated splashes of lukewarm then cool water. A touch of antiseptic lotion on the treated area will help.

Whitehead. A whitehead forms when there is a buildup of oily substance from the sebaceous glands that pushes up to the surface skin. The substance is usually white or yellow in color and needs to be released in order for the whitehead to go away. Hold a wet, warm washcloth on the whitehead. Gently press and the substance should come right out. Avoid purposely breaking the skin that covers the whitehead. Apply antiseptic lotion.

Pimple. A pimple may begin as a blackhead or a whitehead. Because the sebum or oil from the sebaceous glands clogs the pore opening, not allowing it to be released normally, the skin becomes irritated and forms pus around the unwanted clogged area, producing a pimple. Once again, steam your face or hold a warm washcloth on the pimple. This will help the pore to open. Then apply antiseptic lotion or medication. If you're like me, at the first sign of a pimple, you'll want to squeeze it to pieces, praying it will disappear. Please don't do it! If a pimple is not mature, pushing on it will not force anything out. Plus, squeezing will force the infected substance out the bottom of the pore, spreading it to the surrounding area. Also, squeezing can bruise or destroy skin cells, often causing scars to form. So, do yourself a favor—*don't squeeze.*

Acne. Acne is different from pimples. Acne is ongoing, more severe, and is considered a skin disorder or disease that, unfortunately, can be easily identified by its inflamed appearance. People with acne—or any breakout, for that matter—should never be teased. I am sure they are well aware of their problem. If you have acne, seek the medical assistance of a dermatologist. Your doctor can prescribe medicated cleansers, surface antibiotics, or internal antibiotics. Tetracycline and accutane are the most commonly prescribed medications for acne. As with any medication you take, be sure your dermatologist warns you of all possible side effects. Facial scrubs, masks, cleansing pads, and heavy moisturizers should be avoided on acne-prone skin.

Sun and Skin

We can't talk about skin care without mentioning that big fiery red thing up in the sky—the sun. I realize that sunshine provides us with warmth and vitamin D, but when it comes to your skin, the sun is not your friend.

Did you know your skin has a built-in system that tries to protect itself from the harmful rays of the sun? It's called a tan. Exposure to the sun causes your skin to darken and produce more melanin, which serves as a protective covering to prevent or at least slow down the sun's damaging effect on the tissue below.

How can the sun's rays be so bad when they feel so good? Well, damage happens slowly. The extent of damage is determined by your skin type and the amount of overexposure to the sun, but damage occurs because ultraviolet rays break down the collagen (protein) fibers and the delicate elastin tissues of the skin.

Collagen and elastin tissue keep your skin looking young, tight, and nearly wrinkle free. Once these fibers are destroyed, there is next to nothing that can be done about it. Antiwrinkle and collagen creams are limited in their effectiveness.

Oh sure, it's fashionable to have a tan, but years from now it won't be fashionable to be as wrinkled as a raisin! The sun's ultraviolet rays are considered the number-one cause of premature aging. Lines, wrinkles, and pigment spots caused by sun damage can be avoided if you are conscious of the ultimate results.

To tell you to stay out of the sun or even to limit your exposure to the early-morning or late-afternoon hours would be futile. Who goes to the beach at seven o'clock in the morning? So, at least let me give you some good, solid hints to follow while you have fun in the sun.

Sunshine Do's

Do wear a sunscreen with an SPF (Sun Protection Factor) of 8 or 10 when you first begin to work on a tan. An SPF of 2 allows you to stay in the sun twice as long as you could if you had no protection. An SPF of 8 allows you to stay in the sun eight times as long, with less sun damage. Building a good base builds a safer and healthier tan. Reapply sunscreen after swimming or perspiring.

Do be patient. The tanning process is slower but less damaging when you use a sunscreen. As your skin begins to tan, lower your SPF to a 6, then a 4. Four is the lowest! A number 2 does very little.

Do use oil-free, alcchol-free, and fragrance-free sunscreen.

Do wear extra protection between the hours of 10:00 A.M. and 2:00 P.M. when the sun's rays are the strongest. I use an SPF 15 on my eye area. The rest of my face gets an 8 or 10. Facial skin needs the most protection. I also use moisturizer and foundation that contain sunscreen. This is serious business!

Do wear a total sunblock if you are fair skinned, burn easily, or always burn. This skin type is most susceptible to skin cancer.

Do remember that you get sun exposure every day, all year round. Your skin needs constant protection. Make sunscreen part of your daily beauty routine.

Do wear those cute and effective sun visors and wide-brimmed hats to cover your face. Tie a scarf around the base of the hat—one that matches your outfit—for a fun, fashionable look.

Do take advantage of the great-looking sunglasses available. Have

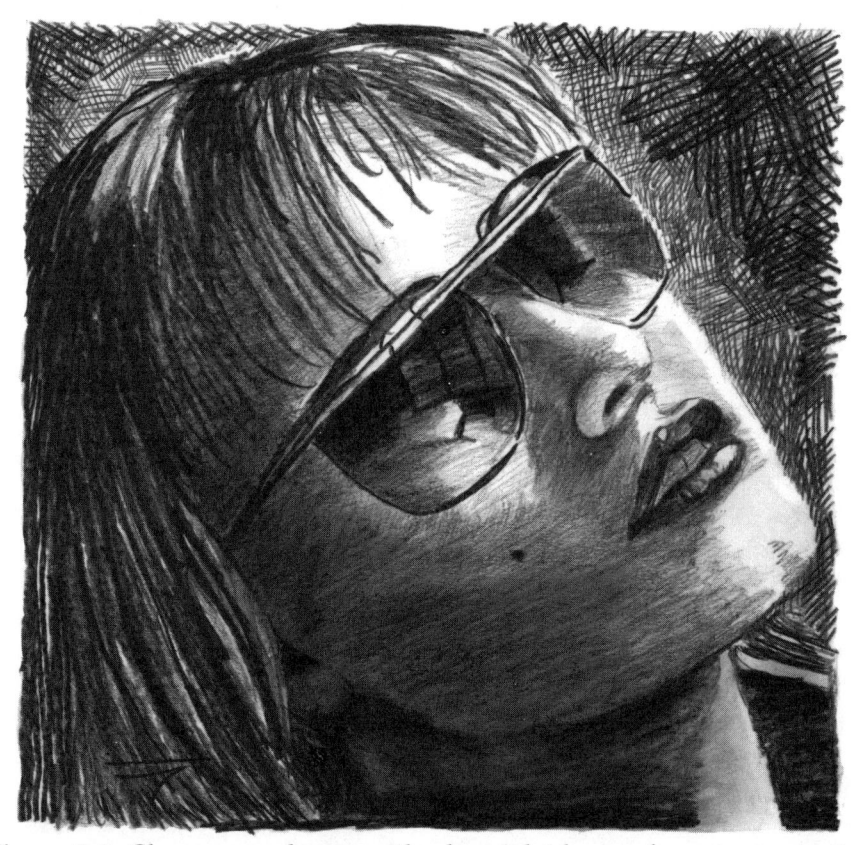

Figure 3-3. Choose sunglasses with ultraviolet lenses for extra protection.

some fun—try lots of colors, shapes, and sizes. Your eyes need dark ultraviolet lenses to really protect them. Select sunglasses with the least amount of frame touching your skin. (*See* Figure 3-3 on page 57.)

Sunshine Don'ts

Don't be fooled. Things that reflect light increase the chance of sunburn—water, sand, concrete, metals, even snow!

Don't forget skin protection on cloudy days. The sun's rays go through clouds, water, lightweight clothing, shade, and those big, beautiful beach umbrellas.

Don't wear cologne or perfume in the sun—you might end up with a spotted tan.

Don't sunbathe if you are taking medication. Consult your doctor first.

Don't forget to apply sunscreen to your neck and the backs of your hands—this will slow wrinkles and pigment spots in later years.

Don't use tanning beds or sun lamps. Both are damaging to the skin. I know salon owners will tell you tanning beds are safe—don't believe them. Ask your dermatologist for a professional opinion.

Don't be lazy about following the do's and don'ts. The result will be prettier, healthier skin.

Using sun protection should prevent sunburn. But should you forget to put it on or overdo exposure to the sun, here's how to cool off a hot burn. Soak in a tub filled with cool water. Then pat your burned skin with a washcloth dipped in apple cider vinegar. This helps remove the sting! Generously apply vitamin E ointment or aloe vera gel. Then, don't burn your skin again!

A severe sunburn may cause the skin to bubble up or blister. Extra care may be needed. Consult your doctor for guidance.

There are sun products on the market you have probably heard of, or maybe even tried. The manufacturers of these products claim they will prepare your skin to produce more melanin when it is exposed to the sun, if used for several days in a row before you plan on sunning. These tan accelerators are to be used *with* your normal sunscreen.

Self-tanning lotions are thought to be better for the skin than actual sun exposure. These lotions change skin tone without damaging the skin's structure. I would suggest using a high-quality self-tanning product. You must be thorough when applying self-tanner. For best results, use your fingers to apply and blend carefully on the ankles, knees, fingers, toes, and face. Use it lightly. You can always reapply but you cannot remove a mistake or an orange tone. The less you use, the more natural it will look. If you use self-tanning lotion remember that when you go in the sun, you look tan but have not built a tanning base—so wear your SPF 8 or 10.

Preventing Problems

The key to maintaining your young-looking and well-cared-for skin is prevention. Wrinkled skin may be the furthest thing from your mind, but *now* is the time to be serious about good skin care. This miracle organ called skin does a better job of keeping us looking good when we take care of it. Prevention pays!

SENSATIONAL SKIN

Project Page

1. List three specific functions of your skin._____
   _____
   _____
   _____

2. Using the techniques described in this chapter, what is your skin type? ____normal ____dry ____oily ____combination

3. What are the special characteristics and nutritional needs of your skin type?_____
   _____
   _____

4. Describe the purpose of the following:
   cleanser_____
   astringent_____
   moisturizer_____

5. Make yourself a skin chart. Include your daily beauty routine: cleanser, astringent, moisturizer, and weekly routine: facial steaming, facial scrub, and facial mask.

6. We have all experienced the embarrassment of breakout! Check the things that will help keep breakout under control:

   ____eating French fries and sweets
   ____drinking lots of water
   ____cleansing once a week
   ____keeping hands away from your face
   ____being less stressed
   ____taking vitamins
   ____smoking cigarettes and drinking alcohol
   ____getting plenty of rest

7. We all wear masks of some kind. What masks do you wear before others? Before the Lord? _____
   _____
   _____
   _____

8. Write a prayer asking God to help you remove your masks and to be yourself.

   Dear God,
   _____
   _____
   _____
   _____

   Signed,
_____

4 MODEL STYLE MAKEUP
Techniques Every Teen Should Know

There was a rare sunset that cool evening. Shades of oranges, reds, and yellows brilliantly shone against the blue sky. She stood gazing at its beauty, trying to calm herself with deep breathing. Her excitement was high, her months of beauty treatments were over. Now, in only a few moments, she would be taken to meet the king. What an exciting moment for a young girl. Was she ready?

I am speaking of Esther, a young Jewish girl. She was chosen to appear before King Ahasuerus as a prospective new queen. She had spent a whole year undergoing what the Bible refers to as "beauty treatments and cosmetics for women." When she was at her best, prepared as well as she could be, she was presented to the king. He fell in love with her. Esther became queen and was later used by the Lord to save the Jews from destruction.

Like Esther, we have a King to prepare ourselves for. We are brought before Him every day. His name is Jesus—the King of kings and Lord of lords. Unlike Esther, we surely don't need to spend a year pampering ourselves before we come to King Jesus. We are not trying to win His love; we already have it!

The cosmetics we use today are far different from those Esther used. But just as she needed guidance in proper makeup for her day, we need guidance for the makeup we wear. The how-to's we will talk about in this chapter are basic and beauty enhancing. I will not be sharing "trendy" techniques or suggestions that will soon change as styles change.

Adding a touch of color here and a bit of emphasis there can give your appearance bright expression and a new glow. The basic and simple techniques you are about to learn can be easily worked into your schedule. They are direct and quick to apply.

As you begin to wear makeup, please be consistent. Show the world a similar face each day. Of course there will be times you will not want to wear makeup at all. You don't want to become a slave to your shadows and blushes, but it's good to make an effort to look your best. Find the look that complements you the most, the techniques that come easiest to you, and use them.

William Shakespeare made the observant statement that God gives us one face and we make ourselves another. Some girls try to do just that. Using cosmetics to hide behind or to alter your facial features are not good reasons for wearing makeup. We have all known girls who wear wild-colored eye shadows, thick eyeliner, pasty-looking foundation—just to make a statement! Other girls wear makeup hoping it makes them look and feel grown up. If a girl is too young, wearing makeup makes her look as if she is playing dress-up.

Each girl matures differently, but a good time to begin your makeup experience is in your late junior high or early high school years. That does not mean you have to appear each day with a full-blown makeup job! And if you don't want to wear it at all until later in life, it's your choice! One piece of advice: Discuss it with your parents first.

I wanted to look like those older girls when I was a young sixth-grader. My mom said *no* makeup at all. One day our family was at K-Mart and I spied a lonely-looking rosy blush lying in a sale basket for just fifty cents! The loose change in my pocket burned as I heard my mom's firm "no makeup" in the far corners of my mind. But only fifty cents? The ornery side of me won out and I dashed to the checkout line to pay for my first and very own blush! I shoved my treasure into my purse, thinking I had put one over on my mom. But no way. Moms are smarter and wiser than eleven-year-old girls.

One day, soon after my big purchase, my mom picked me up from school and guess what she saw? Blush on my cheeks! I had forgotten to wipe it off. I had to learn the hard way that sneaking never pays off and that Mom knows best. I really did look like a little girl, all dressed up with nowhere to go. The rosy blush decorating my cheeks needed to wait a few more years!

Enhancing Your Appearance

The best reason for wearing cosmetics is to enhance your individual appearance. You won't find a chapter full of corrective techniques here! Corrective makeup techniques were designed to give all faces the illusion of being oval shaped. How ridiculous. There is no perfect face shape that we need to try to imitate. Your face shape and special features are already perfect because they're from God.

Way Bandy, who is a respected and talented makeup artist, says in his book *Designing Your Face* that the question of face shapes is unfitting for today's woman. He makes the point that each person's bone structure is an individual matter and that each face has a beauty potential all its own. Beauty cannot be based on any so-called norm such as an oval face shape.

The Natural Look

Makeup techniques that supposedly correct are not valid in light of our God-designed faces. Techniques that enhance are. Enhancing your features, while keeping a natural look, will give the best appearance and make the best statement.

The natural look is soft and pretty. Lighter tones and matching colors allow *you* to be noticed rather than your makeup. Girls on magazine covers and in cosmetic ads, television soap opera stars, and fashion show models often wear what I call fashion makeup. They use too much color and exaggeration. They make themselves look unnatural and unreal. That look may work for their purpose, but that is not our goal.

The natural look lets you put your best face forward! It also allows your outer appearance to be an expression of the inner person Jesus wants you to be, having a gentle and peaceful nature. Soft and natural on the outside, soft and natural on the inside!

The techniques and colors I share with you will help you look your best . . . naturally.

Building a Base

On freshly cleansed skin lay the groundwork for a pretty new look, beginning with base or foundation. (*See* Figure 4-1 in the color section.) This will even out your skin tones by giving a unity of color to your face. Foundation also serves as a gentle shield, protecting your skin from wind, dirt, and humidity. It will even give your skin a smoother appearance.

Foundation comes in several forms. Creams and liquids give a glowing look to dry or normal skin. Cake, dual (double purpose) powder, and water-base foundations give a shine-free look to oily skins. The most recent innovation in foundation is mousse, suitable for all skin types—especially for those who are brave and daring! I recommend oil-free or water-based foundations. These let your skin breathe and help to prevent possible breakout from oil blockage.

To select a foundation that is right for you, match it directly to your skin color and skin type. Test foundation color along your jawline, not on your wrist or the back of your hand. If there is not a tester available, hold the bottle against your skin and check it out in a mirror. This is harder to match, but do your best. The color that is the closest wins! You may find, as I often do, that I need to blend two foundations together to get the shade I need.

If you have a very light skin tone, try a color one shade darker. Blend carefully.

Prefoundations are designed to even out skins that have a reddish or yellowish cast to them. These are unnecessary for most skins. Using a true beige foundation seems to work just as well.

When you are applying makeup, be sure you are in a well-lighted area, such as a bathroom, where water, lights, a towel, and a mirror are readily available. These are especially helpful in making sure your foundation is well blended.

In applying foundation, pour a penny-sized dot on your index and middle fingers. Then rub some on the index and middle fingers of your other hand and gently apply to your entire face, being extra careful to blend on your eyelids, under eye, hairline, jawline, and nostril areas. (*See* Figure 4-3 in the color section.) Oh, and don't forget your lips! A triangular cosmetic sponge helps to blend and press the foundation onto your skin (*See* Figure 4-4 in the color section.) Sponges are another way to apply foundation. Use the quick patting movement or press-and-release method called "stippling." Be sure the foundation is light and even. You want to avoid a "heavy" look.

You don't need foundation on your neck. Just feather the foundation along your jawline using a sponge, tissue, or towel. If you have selected the proper shade, the color of your face and neck area should be the same. Turn your head to the side and look in the mirror to check this.

Foundation makes breakout less noticeable. I'm sure you have already found that out. For increased coverage, after you have powdered your face, simply dot more foundation on the breakout, then powder that spot again. (*See* Figure 4-2 in the color section.) Now, quit worrying about it!

You may choose to skip foundation altogether. Most young skins do not need it. To get the same benefit of foundation without using it, brush on a light layer of powder that is the same color as your skin tone. This will even out your skin tone and give your face a smooth appearance.

Face Sculpting

Just as an artist would add light and dark tones to a portrait on a canvas to give it a three-dimensional, lifelike appearance, so you can add similar shades to your face to create interest. This technique is called *contouring*.

Contouring looks most natural when you do it with foundations or air-spun powder-cream products. You can also use shaded powders. Please note, this step is optional and can look fake on young faces!

To highlight, contour with a foundation a few shades lighter than your regular one. This will bring out areas you want to emphasize. Highlight under your eyes, extending from the inner corner of your eye along the top of your cheekbone, back toward your hairline. (*See* Figure 4-5 in the color section.) Using your finger or a sponge, blend the lighter color very thoroughly. You don't want raccoon-looking eyes! Using light shades, you may want to contour the center of your forehead, your lower jaw, or areas that naturally have shadows. For some faces this would be the inner corners of the eyes, creases of the nostrils, or the dip between the lower lip and chin. Keep your highlighting very subtle and well blended.

Contour with a foundation a few shades darker under the cheekbone to give a rounded appearance to the cheek area. Simply blend the darker tone from the ear area along the under part of the cheekbone, slanted downward to the center of the face. Stop even with the center or outer edge of the eye. It sounds complicated, but I want you to have it on right!

Like the highlighting, darker shades

should be very subtle and well blended. You don't want your face to look muddy.

Contouring takes practice, and you should try it out in private before you appear with it on in public!

Powdered Perfection

Powder is used to absorb excess oil. It sets the foundation and minimizes pore size, giving your skin a polished appearance. Powder also sets the stage for your eye shadows and blushes to be applied with ease.

Powder is available in two forms: loose and pressed. Loose powder gives a light dusting layer; pressed powder can leave a cakelike look to your skin, depending on what you use to apply it with. Often a puff pad or cotton ball can leave your powder looking too thick. A big fluffy brush dipped in loose powder and lightly tapped against the container to shake off excess allows you to apply the right touch to your face. Using light strokes, brush powder over your entire face, including your eyelids. (*See* Figure 4-6 in the color section.) Quick and easy! I use loose powder at home and carry pressed powder with a brush applicator in my purse.

Translucent or colorless powder is best. It allows the foundation or your natural skin tone to show through. Skin-toned powder can replace foundation. Also, light or dark powder can be used to contour, after you use a translucent tone. Translucent powder is too light for dark skins. Use powder that is the same tone as your skin.

Colored powders can add a soft glow to your skin. Those with a touch of fine glitter are dashing for evening wear or fun in the sun.

Expressive Eyes

Eyes are full of expression! They send messages and tell stories that we sometimes are not even aware of. Emotions such as love, joy, sadness, fear, and kindness are all expressed through our eyes. Eyes allow us to look around us, taking in all sorts of information. Eyes are an important means of communication!

What do you communicate with your eyes? You have heard the expression "If looks could kill." These are eyes that show sharp hatefulness. Puppy-dog eyes show innocence and warmth. Eyes of love are gentle eyes sending messages of acceptance, kindness, and caring.

In Proverbs 6:17 the Bible tells us of a certain kind of eyes the Lord hates. These are eyes that show haughtiness. Haughty eyes are selfish eyes that are full of evil pride. Haughty eyes seem to give a false importance to the person showing them, making you feel worthless. A person with haughty eyes usually has a hard heart. Note: You *choose* to show haughty eyes!

The Lord desires softhearted children who will replace haughty eyes with eyes of love. Eyes of love do not judge or put others down. They show approval, forgiveness, and gentleness. They are eyes that belong on the one who loves the Lord and seeks to please Him.

The way we apply makeup to our eyes can add a look of softness, not haughtiness, to them. The soft, natural look will complement your love-expressing eyes!

Eyeliner

The purpose of eyeliner is to define your eyes and make your lashes look fuller. Therefore, line your eyes with colors similar to your eyelashes such as brown, brown-black, gray, or soft charcoal. Lining with blues, greens, violets, or other bright shades doesn't give a natural look.

Lining can be done with eyeshadow, using the edge of the applicator to get a thin line. Apply directly against your lashes. Another way to line is to use a soft kohl pencil. This is probably easier. Always smudge the liner with a smudge-tip, sponge, cotton-tip, or your finger. This gives it a softer look. You want to avoid a hard, distinct line.

Placement of the eyeliner is simple. Guiding your pencil along your lashes, begin at the outer corner of the eye, working under the lower lashes. The outer corner will be the thickest place. As you move toward the inner corner, the line should gradually become thinner. About three-fourths of the way in, blend the pencil line with your lash line so it is not obvious where the line ends. (*See* Figure 4-7 in the color section.)

Lining along the top is done the same way. Begin at the outer corner of your eye, thin the pencil line, and blend it in with your lashes near the inner corner. Smudge! Connect liner at the outer corner.

If your eyes are moist, causing your liner to run off during the day, simply apply an extra layer of translucent powder directly under your lower lashes before applying the liner.

Always line your eyes around the outside rather than on the inner lid directly next to your eyeball. This makes your eyes look larger and more honest. Lining on the inner lid gives a closed look to your eye. It also forces the liner into your eye duct. This is not healthy for your eye.

Eye Shadow

Eye shadow brightens your eyes and adds interest to them. To focus attention on your eyes, use neutral-colored shadows! Using blue, green, lavender, and other bright colors takes away from your natural eye color. These shadows cause others to notice your makeup rather than your eyes!

Warm skin tones will need eye shadows ranging from ivory to peaches to browns. Cool skin tones look best with a range from pinks to bright burgundies to mauves. (*See* the chapter on color for a further explanation of warm and cool skin tones.)

Save frosted shadows for highlighter in the evening. Use matte or frost-free shadow for day wear. Follow this simple three-step process for eye shadow application (*see* Figure 4-8):

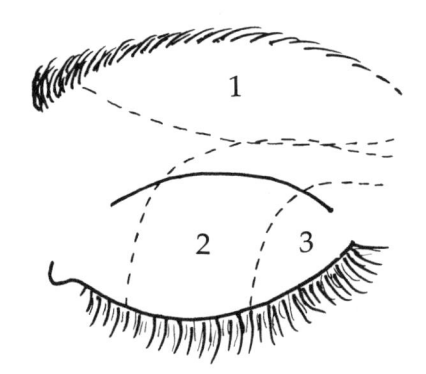

Figure 4-8. Apply eye shadow where specified.

1. Apply an ivory or pink highlighter over the entire lid from lashes to eyebrow. Never use white. (*See* Figure 4-9 in the color section.)

2. Apply a medium-toned shadow

three-quarters of the way across the lid, leaving the inner one-quarter showing the highlighter color. Extend the shadow toward the end of your eyebrow—sort of a faint wing-tip effect. Blend. (*See* Figure 4-10 in the color section.)

3. For extra depth, mostly for evening, add a darker shadow on the outer one-quarter of the lid and into the crease area. Blend so that no obvious line shows.

So many girls want to shadow or line their eyes with bright greens, blues, or lavenders. These colors can be used as accents on the outer corner of the eye next to the liner. Use powder shadows for this. Avoid getting the accent too thick.

Don't waste money purchasing multicolored shadow compacts. Many times you can only use one or two of the colors that are included. If you find one that is full of the perfect colors for you, great. Just be selective. Single shadows are more practical for most of us.

Several companies have put out "pick your own" compacts. You can select the individual colors you want to put in them. These make more sense!

Eyelashes

Mascara makes the eyes! Choose brown or brown-black. Black is used with very dark hair or dark skin tones. Blonde-haired girls should avoid black mascara because it can make them look hard. Colored mascaras look unnatural. Save them for crazy occasions or costume parties.

Mascara should be fragrance free and easy to remove. Waterproof types usually contain an acrylic substance that should not be near your eyes!

To remove mascara use oil-free, fragrance-free eye makeup remover. Read the labels!

To apply, use the tip of the mascara wand to coat the ends of each lash. (*See* Figure 4-11 in the color section.) Let dry. Go back through your lashes, covering them with mascara from the root to the tip. Be sure to twirl the wand as you apply the mascara. This keeps it from drying out in one spot. Apply two coats and don't forget your bottom lashes. Tip your chin down and look up into the mirror to apply mascara to your bottom lashes. Come up just underneath them.

Sharing makeup, especially mascara, with your friends can spread bacteria. Try to remember to keep your makeup touch-up kit with you so you won't be tempted to share. Replace your mascara every six months to keep it sanitary.

If your eyelashes are sticking together, separate them with an old toothbrush or eyelash comb. Please, do not use a pin! If your lashes are sticking because your mascara is too thick and gloppy, throw your mascara away and buy a new one!

Getting mascara on your skin can be a real hassle. Touch the smear with a damp cotton-tip. Twirl the end of the cotton-tip to avoid further smearing. Do not rub it off!

In most cases, eyelash curlers are only necessary for lashes that grow straight out. Be gentle with your lashes when you use a curler. Don't pull or squeeze too hard. Check your lashes from the side to be sure there are no sharp angles.

Eyebrows

If you stand six to eight feet away from a mirror wearing no makeup, can you see all of your eyebrow? If you can see only the first half of it, you are a prime candidate for eyebrow powder.

Most eyebrows get thin near the ends and need an extra boost. The eyebrow serves as a frame for your eye. Nobody wants half a frame.

Using a stiff slanted-edge brush, add shadow beginning at the arch area of your eyebrows. Brush the powder downward, ending evenly at the lowest part of your eye shadow. This will complete your eye look. (*See* Figure 4-12 below.)

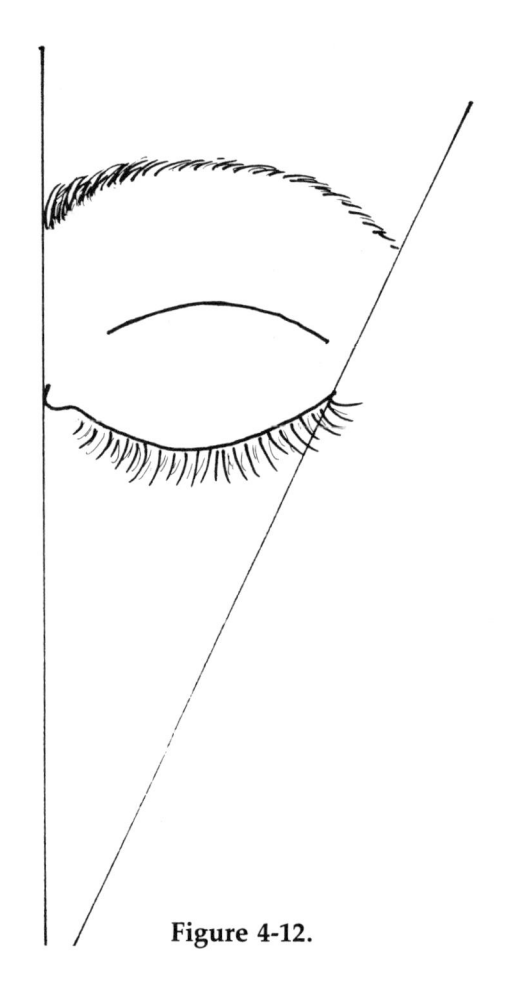

Figure 4-12.

Eyebrows add expression. High-arched brows give a bright, surprised look. A straight brow gives a concerned look. Eyebrows can be shaped to give the expression you desire. I recommend that you go with your natural arch, that is, keeping the highest point of your eyebrow right where it is.

Plucking a few strays is not a bad idea for keeping your brows looking clean. Pluck in the direction of your hair growth to avoid extra pain. Your eyes will probably water the first several times you tweeze your brows. Try pressing an ice cube on your skin before tweezing if you just cannot take the sting.

The best time to tweeze is before your shower or before bedtime. Let the redness fade before applying makeup. Be sure to check for strays and new growth every other day. Your eyebrow should begin even with the inner corner of your eye, arch, then end near the other corner of your eye. (*See* Figure 4-12.)

Keep eyebrows combed upward. To make them stay, put a touch of hair spray on your brow brush and comb through your brows.

Cheery Cheeks

Everyone has been in embarrassing situations. Ever had a chair pulled out from under you? Your shirt on inside out? A price tag still attached to your new dress when you wore it to school? Discovered that a very important zipper was unzipped? Life's little surprises can be embarrassing, and embarrassing moments cause us to blush. When someone tells you that you're blushing, it means your face is turning a rosy color. It's natural. The increased flow of blood rises to the skin surface, giving you sudden color.

The cosmetic "blush" was given its

name because it imitates the natural blushing process.

Blush adds a soft radiance of color to your face. It emphasizes your cheekbone area and centers more attention around your eyes, making you look alive and fresh!

Here again, the name of the game is natural. A light dusting of powder blush that is well blended on the edges will give you the winning look.

Blush is applied in the same places that fill with color when you blush naturally: your cheeks, the edges of your forehead, chin, and sides of your neck.

Look into a mirror. Put three fingers on your cheekbone. What direction do your fingers take? Downward, upward, straight back, circular, or triangular? An upward slant! This is the best direction to apply blush, directly on the cheekbone in an upward slant toward your hairline. As a general rule, blush should not be applied to your cheeks any lower than the end of your nose, and no farther toward your nose than the center of your eye. (See Figure 4-13.)

The tint of your blush will depend upon your skin tone and hair color. Warm skin tones with yellow-blonde to auburn-red hair look best in pink-peach, true peach, coral, or ginger-toned blush. Cool skin tones with hair color in the range of ash blonde, brunette, or black use pretty pinks, rose, or mauve. Dark skins are best complemented with deep rose or burgundy-plum-tinted blush.

Light-toned skin needs a light-toned blush. Medium-toned skin needs medium tones. The less contrast there is between your skin tone and blush intensity, the more appealing your appearance will be.

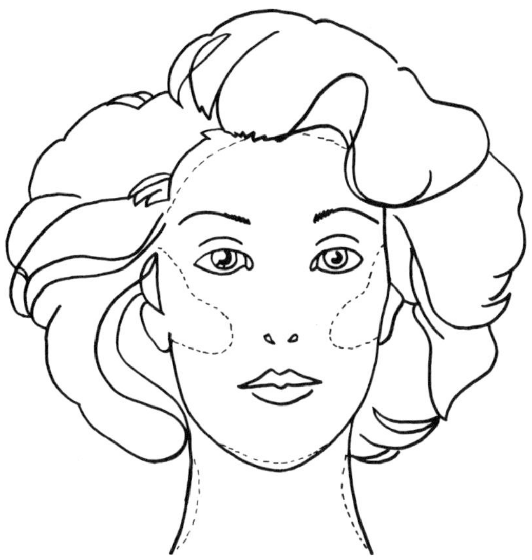

Figure 4-13. Blush Application Guidelines

More and more cosmetic companies are supplying tester units in stores so customers can select a blush tint more accurately. Take advantage of testers, but use a bit of caution. To prevent contacting or spreading germs, use a tissue to wipe off the sample blush that's in the tester unit. Now use a clean tissue to apply the blush to your cheek. Do not use the blush brush that is in the tester unit. The same holds true for eye shadows and lip color testers. Be safe and sanitary! You might even test the blush by holding the blush-smeared tissue next to your skin to see if it's the perfect match.

To apply your powder blush, brush the blush with the applicator, then tap off the excess. Using light, even strokes, start next to your hairline and work toward your nose. (See Figure 4-14 in the color section.) Control the amount and intensity of the blush. If you get too much, dust translucent powder over the blush area. This is also a great way to blend the edge of your blush. My, how lovely you look!

If you apply blush to your forehead,

chin, and neck, be sure you do it very subtly, much lighter than your cheeks. This especially holds true on your neck. If you are wearing a shirt with a collar or high neckline, skip the blush on the neck! No need to get blush on your clothes.

Wearing your blush in these particular places gives a complete look. A little color in these specific spots causes another person to notice your entire face rather than just your cheek and eye area. Blush on the end of your chin visually separates your face from your neck. You may want to try a touch of blush on top of your eyeshadow. It's a nice effect.

I have mentioned only powder blushes because they are the easiest to work with. They are also better for your skin than creams or gels. Powder blushes are applied on your skin surface; creams, liquids, and gels are rubbed into your skin. Gels actually stain your skin and should be avoided completely.

Frosted or iridescent blushes do not look as natural as those with a matte finish (nonfrosted). Oily skins especially should steer clear of sparkly cosmetics. As skin matures, frosted makeup makes lines and wrinkles more noticeable.

Contouring can be done with blushes, using a two-toned combination. For example, use rose blush under your cheekbone and pink on your cheekbone. I personally prefer to contour with my foundations.

Lovely Lips

Lips are definitely one of our attention-getting features! We tend to look at lips as people talk to us. Like eyes, lips can tell a lot about a person. Tightly pursed lips usually do not spread good news and happy endings the way a smile does. The loveliest-looking lips are the lips that are smiling.

Lip products come in a variety of sizes and shapes. You can choose from retractable sticks, pencils, slim sticks, pot gloss, and tube gloss with an applicator.

Consistencies include matte or noncreamy lip cosmetics, creamy moisturizing types, semigloss that feels smooth, or gloss that leaves your lips with a silky feel. Heavy lip covers don't let any of your natural lip color shine through the way some glosses do. However, use glosses lightly. Too much gloss looks drippy wet!

Most lip products can be applied directly, but some need an applicator. Fingers are the most convenient lip tools, but lip brushes work better and don't leave your fingers messy. Lip brushes should be soft and pliable to give a smooth, even look to your lips. Brushes are not hard to use.

Lip liners are used to define your lips and to help keep glosses from spreading onto your surrounding skin. They come in pencil style and are waxy, like a crayon. If you choose to use a liner, the color must match your lipstick or gloss. I do not line my lips on a regular basis. To me, liners are simply not necessary. I can get a nice line by using the preformed edge of my lipstick. Simply glide the edge of your stick along the outer edge of your lips. For a sharper line and a truer color from your lipstick, cover your lips with a thin layer of foundation before applying liner and color.

Selecting the best lip color for you will depend on your skin tones. First you need to determine if you have warm or cool skin tones. Cool tones will need lip colors in the pink-rose family. Warm skin tones will look best in the peach family. Choose a color that harmonizes with your blush and eyeshadow. All color used on your face and nails should match. This is the secret to a truly natural and pretty appearance.

Avoid unnatural tones like orange, brown, yellow, black, blue, white, and purple on your lips. Just because they are available does not mean they should be worn. They might be great for a Dracula movie, but not for your lips!

Lip color will always look better if it is on the lighter side. Dark lips look small and attract attention away from other areas. The soft, gentle look of lighter shades is more appealing. If you can't find that perfect shade, try mixing two shades together. For an added touch of sparkle, put some frosted gloss in the center of your lips. (*See* Figure 4-15 in the color section.)

When you aren't wearing lip cosmetics, your lips still need attention. Like your skin, your lips need to be moisturized. Chapped lips are a sure giveaway that you have neglected your lips. They can become rough, dry, and cracked due to wind, sunburn, or lack of oil glands in the lips. When they get chapped you may be tempted to bite or peel off the skin. Don't do it! Keep a tube of Blistex or a lip-balm type of product close at hand. For chapped-lip prevention, put a dab of petroleum jelly on your lips before bedtime. Make this a nightly affair between you and your lips!

Prelipstick conditioners are good for keeping your lips moist. Apply one after your facial moisturizer. This will give it time to work before your lip color goes on. One more ounce of protection and you're all set: Use a lip product that contains sunscreen. This is especially important for days at the beach or on the ski slopes.

One last thing: You may think this sounds ridiculous, but some girls do this, so it needs to be mentioned. Do not use lipstick as a blush! Lipsticks and glosses are not meant for your cheeks. They're too harsh for your facial skin. Keep your lipsticks on your lips!

Lips are the entrance to your mouth. This reminds me of a prayer in the Psalms. David wrote, "Let the words of my mouth and the meditation of my heart be acceptable in Thy sight, O Lord" (Psalms 19:14).

Using your lips to speak words of love, kindness, encouragement, concern, and forgiveness—all acceptable in the Lord's sight—will make your lips lovelier than their shape, shade, or shine.

Pretty as a Picture

The brand of cosmetics and the amount of money you spend on your makeup means very little. In many cases it is true that you get what you pay for. In choosing cosmetics, the quality is important, but the colors you choose are just as important. Though I recommend investing in quality skin-care products, makeup products in a less expensive line are usually just as good as the expensive ones. Do some comparison shopping before you buy. Your color coordination is what makes your look, not the brand of blush or lip gloss you are wearing.

You may have noticed that I have not mentioned much about variety of makeup styles. I believe in one face for all occasions. Sure, you can vary things a little. Adding more color for evening or brighter shades for daytime is great. The techniques and placement, however, do not change.

Makeup colors will automatically match your wardrobe if you wear colors that harmonize with your natural skin tones—cool or warm. If you wear an outfit from the opposite color family, tone down your blush, eye shadow, and lip color. This way you won't clash!

For that *complete* makeup look, use cosmetics in the order given. For makeup on the run, try this quick combination: powder, medium-toned eye shadow, mascara, light blush, and a hint of lip color. That should do it when you are in a big rush! Always remember, as a final step in your makeup routine, check for lines that might need softening and colors that need to be blended.

Following these techniques and color guidelines will help you achieve a natural look—the look that lets the true you shine through. (*See* Figure 4-16 in the color section.) Keep it light, keep it natural, and keep it pleasing to the eyes of others and to the eyes of the Lord.

MODEL STYLE MAKEUP

Project Page

1. Esther prepared herself for King Ahasuerus. How does prayer and reading the Bible prepare us for our King, Jesus? _____
   _____
   _____
   _____

2. Why is it important that your makeup give you a natural look?
   _____
   _____
   _____

3. Pull your hair back and take a picture of yourself wearing no makeup. Now, give yourself or have a friend give you a makeover following the directions given in this chapter. When you are finished, style your hair and take another picture. Compare your before and after photos.

4. Eyes are full of expression. What do your eyes express? _____
   _____
   Look into a mirror. Use a piece of paper to cover your nose and mouth. Now practice using your eyes to express the following: happiness, concern, love, laughter, compassion, anger, surprise.

5. According to your skin tones, what shades of makeup are best for your:
   eyes_____
   cheeks_____
   lips_____
   nails_____
   eyelashes_____

6. If you have been wearing blues, greens, purples, or similar bright shades on your eyelids, try using them as accent colors instead. See if your friends notice the difference.

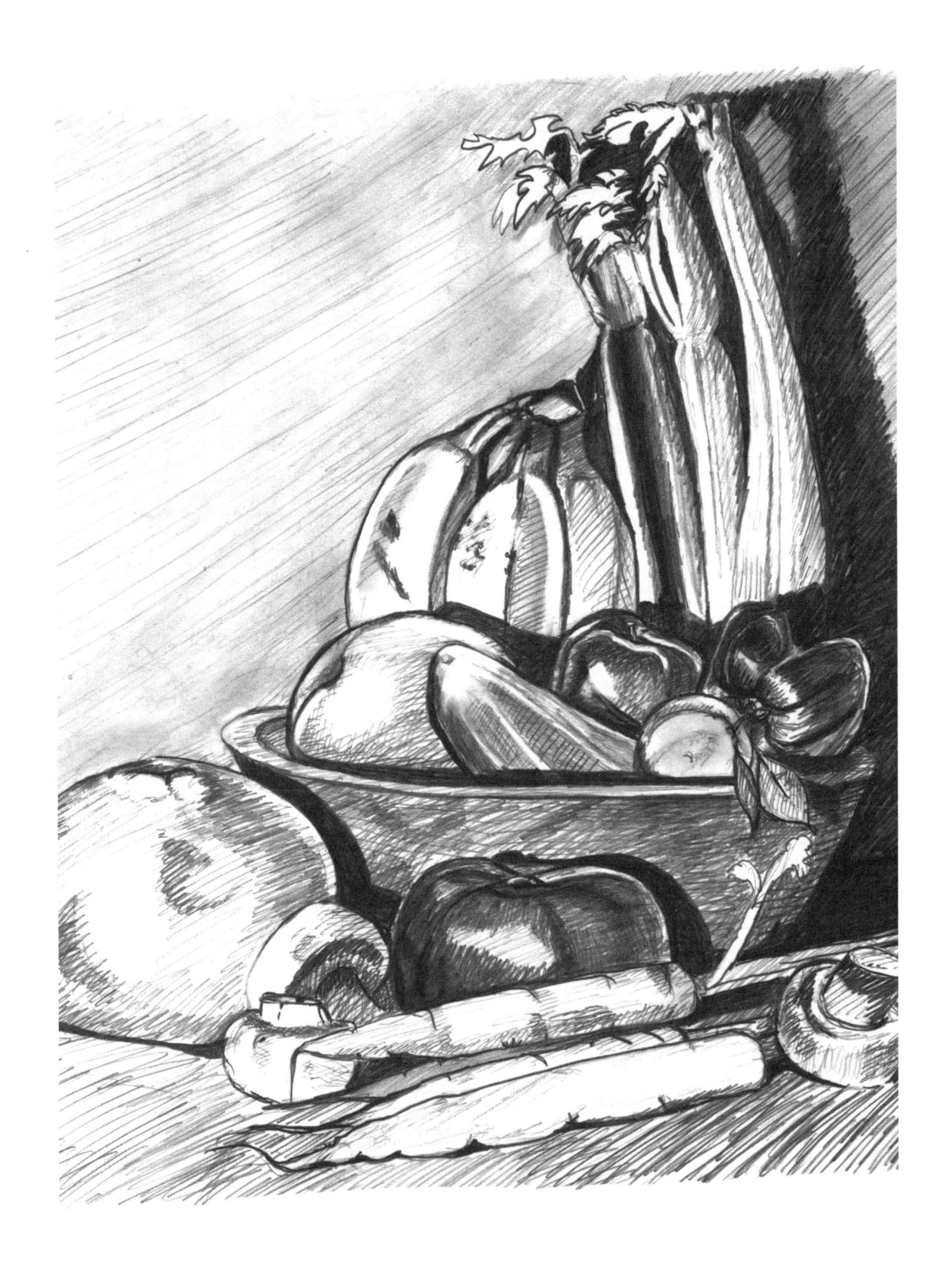

5 NUTRITION
Building a Better Body

"Oh, no," you're probably saying. "Here comes another lecture on what I should eat and what I shouldn't eat. I'll bet she'll even tell me to cut out sugar and eat more fruits and vegetables!"

Well, if that's what you're thinking, you are right on both counts. I *am* going to tell you which foods are best for you, and I *am* going to tell you to ease up on that sinfully sweet sugar! I'm even going to tell you, "Yes, the rumor you've heard so many times is true: You *are* what you eat!"

What you eat will be evident in the appearance of your skin, hair, nails, and figure. What you eat has a lot to do with lasting physical beauty.

What you put into your body will also determine how well it operates. If you put water in your gas tank instead of gasoline, your car won't run. Even if you put in regular gas when your car needs super unleaded, it won't run as well. "But a car is a machine," you say, "not a person." True, but your body is a machine too. If you fill it with gooey doughnuts, candy bars (do Snickers really satisfy you?), bags and bags of chips or supersalty snacks, don't expect your body to feel good and perform at its best. It has to be cared for if it is going to operate effectively and if it's going to have lasting beauty.

In this chapter I want to talk about dieting, figuring out how much you should weigh, eating habits, balanced eating, sensible weight gain and loss, reasons for eating, and how drugs and alcohol affect your beauty program.

The Feared Four-Letter Word: Diet

I'm going to diet; I should diet; tomorrow I'll diet. The whole world is on a diet! When we hear that dirty word *diet*, we think of all the things we can't eat instead of the things we can. We make dieting seem like a punishment. It doesn't have to be negative! All the word *diet* really means is the combination of foods we eat—in other words, the food program we are on.

When a teenage girl asks me if she should go on a diet, my first reaction is to say no. Many girls complain that they are fat or overweight. Most of them are not. They just need to cut out sweets, late-night buttery popcorn, and pizza pig-outs. Then they need to get off their behinds and exercise! A growing young woman should go on a diet only after she has cut down on junk foods and increased her physical activity.

If you are concerned about your weight, pray about it, then talk it over with your parents and go see your family doctor. If your doctor agrees that you could lose a little weight, let him put you on a program. He should monitor your medical condition and progress as you go. Don't do it alone.

Too many girls who think they are fat and unattractive secretly set out to change things. Many of them end up as anorexics or bulimics. Anorexia nervosa and bulimia are eating disorders that are common among girls who are obsessed with weight loss.

Anorexia victims usually starve themselves; bulimia victims overeat and then make themselves vomit. Both may take laxatives, water pills, and diet pills. Usually these girls have a low self-image. Both anorexia and bulimia produce serious health problems that can be lifelong.

Where does this obsession to be thin come from? It comes from our own society, which blasts us with billboards, TV commercials, and magazine ads that try to convince us thin is in. Years ago, just the opposite was true. Larger women were considered more desirable. Just look at some of the old masters' paintings of women. All of them are curvy, round, and buxom! Don't accept the world's message on what is ideal weight. Besides, your body shape and size have nothing to do with your value as a person!

A skinny body has never solved anyone's problems or brought inner happiness. Only the Lord can do that. No problem is too big for God. If you find yourself trapped in the vicious cycle of weight loss and weight gain, go to God for help and share your struggle with your parents or family doctor. You don't have to struggle alone.

If you feel that your friends, or some guy you are wild over, would like you better if you were thinner (or heavier, for that matter), then perhaps you need to get yourself some new friends or a new boyfriend!

The pressures of looking good are high in our society. Dieting is not always the answer. Any food program you are on should be monitored. Have your parents or a friend know what you are doing so they can encourage you. Be realistic about your weight goals. Look at your weight from all angles!

How Much Should I Weigh?

Several factors affect the answer to this question. Weight is a very individual matter. The weight that is right for me may not be right for you. Consider these:

1. *Height.* The taller you are, the more weight your body needs and can hold effectively. The shorter girl will usually want to hold less weight. There are standard charts that suggest a desired weight according to height. I find these charts limiting. Many of them don't take bone structure and muscle weight into consideration. They merely put pressure on us, making us think we are too heavy or too thin. Besides, it's not how much you weigh but how you look that counts!

2. *Bone structure.* Psalms 139:15 suggests that your bone structure is uniquely yours. As a general rule, your weight will be in proportion to your bone structure—small, medium, or large. It is unrealistic for a large-boned girl to expect to weigh the same as her small-boned friend. It is unnecessary for a small-boned person to weigh the same as a large-boned person.

3. *Age.* Your body develops and matures on its own time schedule. Generally, girls begin to add weight at the onset of puberty. As you grow, your weight usually increases. That's only natural. Your metabolism rate—the rate at which your body burns off calories—is also affected by age and will slow down as you get older.

4. *Muscle mass.* This is the amount of muscle tissue you have developed. This affects your weight because muscle weighs more than fat. This is good, though! You want to have more muscle than fat. More muscle and less fat means a healthier body!

Eating Habits

Our eating habits can affect our bodies. Any of the following habits is a warning sign to you:

1. *Eating in secret.* Why is it we think if no one sees us, the calories won't count? You can't fool your body. It knows every time you sneak.

2. *Cheat eating.* Oh, you know! This is when you are in the process of making cookies but half of the dough mysteriously disappears before those cookies hit the oven.

3. *I only had a salad!* Sure you did, but what was in that salad? Meat, cheese, raisins, croutons, bacon bits, creamy sweet dressing, sunflower seeds, and all of those other high-calorie extras. Be honest with yourself.

4. *Before-dinner snack.* We've all done this. You get so excited about going out to eat that you eat before you go out.

5. *Headfirst!* This is the ol' "head in the refrigerator" habit. You have to taste test everything in sight trying to decide what you want to snack on. Don't forget: It may be going in one end but it will show up on the other!

6. *Convenience wins.* This habit leaves you standing with a spoon in one hand and a can or jar in the other. Why prepare it anyway? Just eat it right out of the container. . . .

7. *Eating anywhere.* This habit usually has us eating more than normal. Munching in front of the TV or while studying or riding in the car will not give you the full pleasure that a sit-down meal will. Eat at the kitchen or

dining-room table. Eating on the run is hard on your digestive system.

8. *Anytime, please.* Eating all morning and late at night are easy habits to get into, but quick, straighten things out before you go any further. Late-night food is usually not followed with exercise; therefore, it turns into fat and unburned calories. Try not eating after 7:00 P.M.

These are habits that can be broken. It's just a matter of making a quality decision. Then begin forming a new habit—healthy and balanced eating.

Balanced Food Program

A balanced diet or food program is the key to receiving the nutrients and vitamins you need for perfect health and glowing beauty. Your goal should never be to become model thin, but to maintain good health. This food program is not necessarily meant for weight loss or gain. It is simply my opinion of the best way to feed your body.

When I say "balanced food program," I mean daily choosing foods from the four food groups: (1) Meats, (2) Milk and Milk Products, (3) Fruits and Vegetables, (4) Breads and Cereals. This program should give you the proper combination and amounts of proteins (12 percent), carbohydrates (58 percent), fats and dairy products (30 percent), which your body needs. To find out how much protein, carbohydrate, and fat are in the food you eat, read the labels. Nearly all foods include this information on the package. You could also pick up a booklet that contains this information at your local bookstore.

Health class, nutrition class, and home economics class all teach balanced eating. Don't blow off this information. Eating foods from each of the food groups, either at each meal or on a daily basis, will result in a healthier you.

The Program

I know that following a strict program is hard. That is why the next two sections are only suggestions. It is not unusual for me to stray from the list, but I make an honest effort to do my best. Yes, I occasionally eat a bag of Whoppers or Almond Roca, but "occasionally" for me means once a month maximum! My biggest nutritional loophole is all the pizzas I love to eat. I'm hooked on those steaming hot, cheesy pepperoni pies!

Here is a list of the *minimum* requirements teens need every day:

Milk. Drink two to four glasses of low-fat, 2 percent, or nonfat milk. Your body doesn't need the extra fats in whole milk. You can substitute a cup of yogurt for a glass of milk. A cup of milk equals half a cup of cottage cheese or 2 ounces of cheese. Avoid processed cheeses. Dairy products are great for vitamins A and D. They also provide the calcium your female body needs.

Fruit. Each day have one citrus fruit or a tomato for your supply of vitamin C. Citrus fruits are oranges, lemons, grapefruit, strawberries, and limes. Also have two to four other kinds of fruit. If it is canned fruit, be sure it is packed in its own juices, not heavy syrup. Fruit supplies your body with the natural sugars that are better than refined sugar.

Vegetables. There are so many tastes and textures of vegetables available to us. Take your pick, but eat three to five veggies a day. Most of them are low in calories, so they make great snacks. I like putting a little melted cheese on my vegetables at dinner time. Try a baked potato topped with meat and cheese for dinner sometime!

Eggs. Three eggs a week is a good amount. Have one at breakfast—poached, scrambled, or fried in a small amount of margarine. Hard-boiled eggs are also great on a salad.

Red meat, seafood, poultry. The protein pals! Have about four to six ounces of meat a day. It is better to have more in the early part of the day than at dinner time. Most meats, especially red meats, are harder for our bodies to digest. Red meats are also high in calories. Prepare meat, seafood, and poultry in the least greasy way. Broil, microwave, boil, and Crock-Pot are the best.

Whole grain bread and cereal. Treat yourself to two to three slices of whole grain bread each day. I say whole grain because it contains the complete nutrients, vitamins, and complex carbohydrates that are absent in white and other breads. Whole grain breads are whole wheat, buckwheat, and rye. The best cereals are also grain type. Sugar cereals may seem much more fun, but grain cereals are for serious health-conscious people like you! If you have to sweeten your cereal, try honey.

Butter or fats. There are hidden fats and oils in lots of foods, and your body really doesn't require much fat intake. Limit yourself to one tablespoon a day. If you use low-calorie margarine or mayonnaise you can have a bit more.

The Plan

Now that you know the minimum requirements for a day, here is a sample easy-to-follow meal plan to help you arrange your foods throughout the day:

Breakfast

½ cup orange juice or grapefruit juice or 1 orange or ½ grapefruit
1 egg prepared without fat
1 slice of toast or ½ English muffin
1 teaspoon butter or margarine
1 cup nonfat milk
or
1 cup hot or cold cereal instead of egg
Use part of your one cup of milk for your cereal.

Lunch

Choose one of the following:

½ cup cottage cheese
1 medium tomato
1 fruit
2 crackers
or
3 to 4 ounces lean meat, fish, or poultry. (If you eat these in a sandwich you add 1 or 2 slices of bread. Try a meat-and-cheese croissant, but preferably on the day you don't have toast for breakfast.)
1 fruit
or, for variation:
a huge garden salad full of veggies . . . add one protein—tuna, chicken, cheese, or egg
1 tablespoon dressing
1 fruit
or, another idea:
1 bowl of soup
2 crackers
1 fruit

Dinner

4 to 6 ounces lean meat, fish, or poultry
2 servings of vegetables
Dinner salad with dressing
1 fruit
1 cup nonfat milk
1 whole grain bread slice or roll
1 teaspoon butter or margarine

Substituting One Food for Another

To keep your eating balanced, you can do some substituting. If I am going to have pizza for dinner, I don't eat bread during the day. The crust makes up for a full day's supply of bread. The cheese and pepperoni count as my protein and dairy products.

If Mexican food is on my mind, the tortillas are in place of bread. I get my protein and carbohydrates from refried beans, meat, vegetables (with lettuce, tomato, onion, and salsa) all wrapped up in my burrito.

This is called substituting. It means planning ahead, but it is worth it to keep your eating balanced. Try it. See if you can calculate your daily needs into your meal planning. The challenge will keep your mathematical and creative thinking sharp!

Delicious Desserts!

Oh my gosh! Can you really have dessert? Yes you can! The key is to be sensible and choosy. A bowl of fresh strawberries, trickled with honey and wheat germ, is a tasty treat after dinner. How about a dish of sugar-free gelatin topped with a tablespoon of whipped cream? Or, this is my dessert delight: two small scoops of vanilla ice milk, polka-dotted with a handful of chocolate chips. Yum!

You can make sugar-free, low-calorie frozen fruit pops using Crystal Light or sugar-free Kool-Aid. Freeze them in cups and put sticks in them. How fun!

Sensible Snacks

The first thing I used to do when I got home from school was run for the kitchen. You probably do the same thing. There is something about getting out of school that makes us hungry. It is probably relief!

When eating that after-school snack, let your brain be your guide, not your taste buds or emotions. A piece of fresh fruit or raw veggies are fabulous snacks. One or two cookies if you must. No fair eating a whole bag of chips in front of the TV. No sugar-filled candy! Drink a full glass of water or juice if you are really starved. The feeling will go away quickly. Remember, you are what you eat. Stay away from those Twinkies and Ding Dongs unless you want to become one!

What to Avoid

Most of us grow up with a sense of right foods and wrong foods to feed a healthy body. Avoid doughnuts, candy, ice cream, cakes, pies, cookies, greasy foods, heavy sauces, gravies, and syrup. The list could go on. These foods will eventually leave your body soft and headed down the road to overweight. I am not saying you can never have these foods, but use wisdom.

Many foods do not need to be avoided, they just need to be prepared properly. Potatoes are wonderfully nutritious. It is the way we fix them or what we put on potatoes that makes them a no-no. French fries, skillet fried, potato chips, and creamy potatoes are not your best choice. However, mashed potatoes and baked potatoes are great. This same principle applies to many other foods.

Meats are another one of those foods that can be abused. Friday-night fish fries or your grandma's country-fried chicken are fine once in a while. Eat them too often and you will feel the effects.

Many foods are available in three forms: fresh, frozen, or canned. Fresh is always best, frozen is next, and canned comes in last. Frozen foods do not have all the additives and preservatives that canned foods do. Yet, fresh is still best.

Calorie Consciousness

I am not encouraging you to become a compulsive calorie counter, but calorie consciousness will work to your benefit when choosing foods. So will keeping count of nutrients. Go to a bookstore and get a calorie-counter book.

Knowing what foods are low or high in calories will tell you what foods you can eat more of and what to eat less of. You will probably be surprised at the calories in many of your favorite foods. Some of the best foods for you, such as fruits and vegetables, are low in calories. Just because a food is low in calories, don't classify it as a diet food.

Another surprise is the difference in the amount of calories in the same food prepared in different ways. For example, one cup of fresh apple is 80 calories. But one cup of sweetened applesauce is 232 calories. Then again, one cup of apple juice is 117 calories. Quite a difference.

If you want to keep track of your calories, do this: For one week write down everything you normally eat (including snacks). Add up the number of calories you consume each day. An average number of calories for a teenager to eat per day is 2100 to 2400. Whether or not you are eating too many calories depends on your body and how fast it burns up calories.

If you want to lose one pound a week, drop 500 calories per day from your total. One pound is 3500 calories. Multiply 500 calories a day times seven days in a week for a total of 3500 calories, or one pound. If you exercise, don't eat less than 1200 calories a day.

If you want to gain one pound a week, add 500 calories a day to your total intake. This works almost every time. Do remember that coupling balanced eating and exercise is the most effective way to go.

Weight Gain: Adding Pounds

Some girls want or need to gain weight. My suggestion is this: Increase the amount of food you eat, but stay within the four food groups. The mistake most thin people make when they want to put on pounds is to go hog-wild eating sweets, milk shakes, or candy. This stuff will make you gain weight, but it will be the wrong kind of weight—you'll add soft fat. Instead, gain solid healthy tissue. Couple your eating with a low-energy activity such as quick walking. This will not make you burn off needed calories but will help you develop good muscle tissue.

Weight Loss: Subtracting Pounds

When losing weight, decrease the amount of food you eat, but maintain a balanced program. Never try to lose more than one or two pounds per week. It just is not realistic or safe. Too many girls set unreachable goals for themselves, then get depressed when they don't reach them.

If you have more than ten pounds to lose, I suggest you go to your family doctor before you start a weight-loss program. Losing too much weight too fast is dangerous. It can mess up your menstrual cycle and digestive system.

Increase the amount of exercise you get when you are trying to lose. This is a must! Exercise is the key to successfully subtracting pounds.

Continue to eat three meals a day, but eat less. Don't think skipping a meal will help. You will only end up eating more at the next meal. Your body will evenly burn off calories if it is fed on a regular basis. Girls who don't eat for a day or two are fooling themselves. When your body has been deprived of food, it will store all the calories you give it next time you eat. You do not end up any further ahead.

Take time to think about what you are eating. Chew, taste, swallow—enjoy! Know when you are full. Then stop eating.

Please beware of crazy fad diets. It seems as if each month every magazine comes out with a new no-fail diet plan. There are water diets, carbohydrate diets, low-protein diets, high-protein diets, and even diets named after famous towns and people. Ignore them!

Never take diet or water pills. They can interfere with your natural body functions. Diet pills claim to curb your appetite, but a large glass of water or juice will do the same thing. Anyway, it isn't always our appetites that need curbing. We do not always eat because we are hungry.

The Whys Behind Our Eating

Often, what we eat is influenced by our emotions or the day's events. For example, try these scenarios on for size: Let's say you have been dating this special guy for six months. Suddenly he decides he wants to break up and says he wants to date around. How do you respond to this crushing news? By crying rivers of tears and eating mountains of food!

Your mother told you to make your bed and wash the dishes before you left the house, but you were rushed and your friends were out in the car honking for you. So you dashed out of the house, bed unmade and dishes unwashed. Your mom grounds you for a week. You feel frustrated, as if you have been treated unfairly. What do you do? Make yourself a huge hot fudge brownie sundae and try to eat your troubles away!

It's Saturday night. Your face broke out on Thursday and no one asked you out for a date. You think it's because all the guys think you are a zit face. So you sit at home, having a pity party and feeling very lonely—and you eat several bags of chips and buttered popcorn while watching the Saturday-night movie.

Do any of these sound familiar? Not all of us are caught in this routine, but most of us can relate at least a little.

Using food to feed your emotions will not solve a thing. It will only cause weight gain and probably make your face break out.

The best way to handle an emotional hunger is through what I call "talk therapy"—not food!

We all need to talk out things that are happening in our lives. We all need to share our thoughts and feelings with someone else. Holding it all in is not the answer. You need a special friend, parent, or youth pastor you can confide in. All of life's situations are easier to handle when you get them "outside" yourself through talking.

If you feel as if you don't have a friend you can share with, remember you do have a friend in Jesus. He is your heavenly Confidant, who is there waiting anytime, anywhere. He wants you to share what is troubling your heart. Go ahead—talk out loud or silently. He can hear you either way. Then be sure you listen quietly for Him to respond!

Emotions and disappointments are best talked through rather than eaten through.

My Personal Story

My personal struggle with weight has had its ups and downs. I am not proud of some weight-loss gimmicks I have tried.

As a teenager I was naturally thin. My friends used to tease me and say that I didn't have a rear end. Of course that wasn't true, it was just that my backside was flat! Being thin never bothered me, though. I liked it. But like many young ladies, I eventually became oversensitive about my weight and body appearance.

By the time college rolled around, I had become extremely weight conscious. One of my friends and I would go on soda-and-cracker diets. I weighed only 112 pounds, but I would try to see how low I could get my weight. At 106 my clothes bagged, but I was happy. I never kept my weight real low—and I would usually gain it back within a few days.

Until college, I had never heard of vomiting as a method of weight control. My good friend Michelle was very thin, yet she was a big eater. She always had bags of candy bars, peanuts, and pastry stashed away in her room. I couldn't figure it out. "Michelle locks herself in the bathroom after she eats and makes herself throw up," Michelle's cousin, Karen, told me one day. "Why?" I asked. "Michelle is obsessed with being thin. I guess she used to be sort of heavy," Karen replied. I was puzzled.

As I got to know more girls at the school, I found out that Michelle was not the only one who did this sort of thing. Being thin, I didn't feel the panic of gaining weight the way some other girls did. I must admit, though, that after I thought vomiting was commonplace, I tried it myself a few times. Vomiting never accomplished anything for me and I was lucky enough not to get hooked on it.

My thinness worked to my advantage when I was a contestant in the Miss Oklahoma Pageant. I won the swimsuit competition and a cash award that I used for college tuition. Not bad for the girl who was nicknamed "bird legs" as a kid.

Just two months after the pageant, I attended a national modeling convention in New York City. I did well and was granted an interview with Wilhelmina Cooper, at that time the owner of Wilhelmina Models, Inc. When she weighed me in her office on that first visit, I was a trim 109 pounds.

I have to be honest and tell you that

it was hard for me to be on my own in New York. Being right in the middle of the beauty world didn't exactly boost my self-confidence. Constantly being compared with other girls and feeling inadequate really made the pressure of modeling very high.

Feeling trapped, I reacted by eating. If I was sad or depressed, I ate. If I felt lonely, I ate. If I was happy and wanted to reward myself, I ate. I was stuck in a vicious cycle. Soon the results of my eating caught up with me. Only four months after I moved to New York I was up to 118 pounds. When I left the Big Apple, I weighed 128 pounds. That was a far cry from 109!

Deciding to move back to Oklahoma was an emotional event. I knew I was doing what the Lord wanted, but at the same time, I became very depressed and continued to eat my way up to 135 pudgy pounds. That may not sound heavy to you, but I am a small-boned person. Needless to say, I didn't feel good about myself, nor did I look good. I felt as if I were carrying around extra baggage that wasn't really part of my body. My shape had changed, no doubt! The weight looked out of place on me. My upper arms were flabby, my waist was almost nonexistent. Most of the weight was in my hip area. With my shoulders still narrow and my hips now wide, I was shaped like a pear. I hated it. That hatred began to turn inward and I developed a serious self-image problem.

Losing weight takes time. It took me years to lose the weight I had gained. I will admit, it was not an easy thing to do. It was a daily struggle. Dieting didn't work for me. Starving myself didn't work. It only made me very sick. Binge eating was not the answer, either.

Because I have been through it, I can honestly tell you that balanced eating, combined with exercise and constant prayer, is the best way to lose weight. The results are longer lasting and better looking.

I could not have lost the weight without the help of the Lord. He supplied me with the hope and self-control I needed. He also helped me see myself as a valuable person, and cured my low self-esteem.

Today my weight has leveled off to a healthy state. I know the weight where my body functions best. I am also much more realistic about my weight, and I no longer panic every time the scale moves up. I know how my body works and what I have to do to maintain my weight. May I also say that the emotional needs I had are now handled much differently. I, too, practice "talk therapy." I take my needs to the Lord in prayer!

I know that in the future my weight and body will continue to change. When I begin having children it will be natural for changes to take place. Also, it is a known fact that as we get older, our metabolism changes. That does not mean we all have an excuse to pork out, but that we will have to continue taking good care of ourselves by eating and exercising right.

Effects of Drugs and Alcohol

Since we are talking about nutrition and caring for our bodies, I want to make you aware of two nutrition and beauty robbers that dance around in costumes of fun: drugs and alcohol.

Drugs and alcohol strip the body of

nutrients and have a lasting effect on skin appearance. Alcohol and cigarette or marijuana smoking age the skin quickly by drying it.

Drugs affect the body in other ways also—many that we are only now discovering. They can alter our thinking, our emotions, and definitely damage our health. Drugs literally invade every part of the body.

Most drugs are addictive. They change the body chemistry, making it dependent upon the drug. Playing with social drugs such as marijuana, cocaine, and crack is not the kind of game you can just walk away from. You must choose to play or not to play. *No one can make you get in the game.*

Alcohol presents the same situation. It is very available but very harmful. *Alcohol is one of the major causes of death among teenagers.* It is nothing to fool around with. Like drugs, alcohol is one of the enemy's tools to destroy healthy young adults.

Most teens experiment with drugs and alcohol because of peer pressure or problems at home. You must decide what your answer to drugs and alcohol will be *before* the question is presented to you. It saddens my heart that many Christian teens wind up in the alcohol-drug trap. They can get out, but it's easier to avoid getting into it if they choose to say no, and then follow through on their decision when the pressure to participate stares them in the face. Choose to respond to the Lord's best rather than the pressure from your friends. Friends? Those who get others trapped in drugs or drinking are not friends.

I honestly believe that drug-and-alcohol use are not pleasing to the Lord. Yes, I know the Scriptures about Jesus turning water into wine and all of that. But seeing the damaging effects of drugs and alcohol on the lives of so many people has convinced me that our loving God wants His children to have no part of this harmful indulgence.

I believe this holds true no matter what your age. I do not believe that once you turn eighteen or twenty-one it is okay to drink. I wish parents who preach to their kids not to drink would get the beer and wine out of the refrigerators and turn the liquor cabinet into a pantry. I know this is not a popular viewpoint, because it makes people uncomfortable.

I urge you to be strong and say no to drugs and alcohol, even if it means losing some friends or having a "straight" reputation. In the end you will win. Just say no. It will do your body a lot of good.

Feeding Your Spirit

We have covered feeding the physical part of us. But what about feeding the other part of us that is equally important—our spiritual self. Yes, that needs nutrition, too. Each of us has a spiritual nature that hungers for God. Some describe it as a God-shaped void that only God Himself can fill.

Many people get wrapped up in the wrong things in their attempts to nourish the spiritual hunger inside of them: cults, wrong spirits, alcohol, drugs, overindulging in TV, movies, or even their jobs. They know they need something, but they can't figure out or admit what their need really is. It is God!

Let's look at a menu for nourishing your spiritual self: The first course you should serve your spiritual hunger is Jesus. Simply ask Him to come and live in your heart. When you do this, you are forgiven and you become one with God and have peace with Him. You are new inside, or born again. Your spirit is what becomes new. And Jesus says in John 6:35 that He is the bread of life and that if we have Him, we will not be spiritually hungry. Just as we don't eat food once and then never again, so we must not fill up once on Jesus and then call it enough! We need to feed on Him daily!

The second course is to be filled with the Holy Spirit. This way you can experience the fruit or the characteristics of the Holy Spirit in your life: love, joy, peace, patience, kindness, goodness, faithfulness, gentleness, and self-control. We have these great qualities in us because Jesus lives in us.

As a third course, serve your spirit the Word of God. This is straight spiritual food that your spirit needs. The Bible is your handbook to life. It teaches you and guides you according to God's will for your life. Jesus said His food was to do the will of His Father God (John 4:34). The same applies to us. It feeds our spirit to learn and to do God's will.

And now for your spiritual dessert! Fellowship. Spending time with other Christians. Finding out what God has done and is doing in the lives of others helps your faith to grow and nourishes your spirit.

You have been beautifully created. You have a physical nature and a spiritual nature. Feeding them both guarantees you complete nutrition.

NUTRITION

Project Page

1. Why is "You are what you eat" a true statement? _____

2. How has society's message of "thin is in" affected most girls' views of themselves? _____

3. Body shape and size do not determine a person's value or worth. What does make a person valuable? _____

4. What are the missing factors in a standard weight chart? _____

5. Make a list of all your bad and good eating habits. Try to think of a way to get each of your bad habits onto the good habits list. _____

6. List three benefits of a balanced food program. _____
_____
_____
_____
_____
_____
_____

Now take a daily inventory to be sure you are eating a balanced menu.
____ meats
____ milk and milk products
____ fruits and vegetables
____ breads and cereals
    ____ 2–4 glasses of 2 percent or nonfat milk
    ____ 2–4 fresh fruits, one citrus
    ____ 3–5 vegetable servings
    ____ 3 eggs per week
    ____ 4–6 ounces meat, seafood, or poultry
    ____ 2–3 slices whole grain bread
    ____ 1–2 tablespoons butter or fat product

7. For one week, keep a chart of all the food you eat—everything. Now get a calorie-counter booklet and add up the number of calories you consumed. You may be over or undereating! To lose one pound per week, subtract 3500 calories from your total. To gain one pound per week, add 3500 to your total intake per week.

8. If you need to cut calories, circle all the sugary or greasy (including chip-type snacks) foods on your chart. Cut those first. Do not cut needed nutrients.

9. Drugs and alcohol have a harmful effect on our bodies. Turn up your creativity level and come up with three ways to say no to drugs and alcohol. _____
_____
_____
_____
_____
_____
_____

Now try them out! Create positive peer pressure. Because you have the courage to say no, you will help someone else have the courage to do the same.

NUTRITION

10. Write a weekly meal plan that will feed your spirit. Include the following courses: Jesus, prayer, Holy Spirit, the Bible, and fellowship with other Christians._____
_____
_____
_____

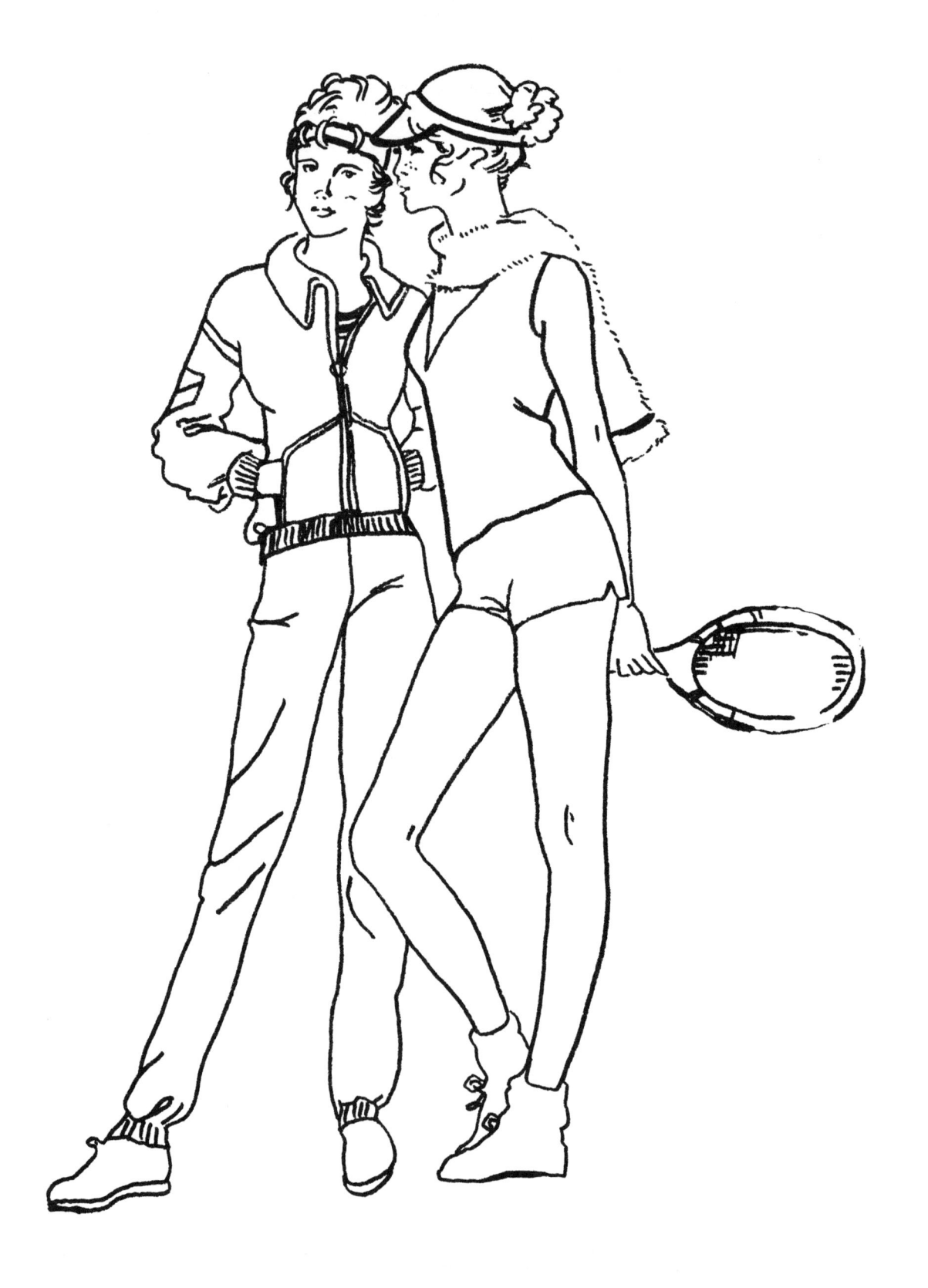

6 TOTAL FITNESS
Just for the Fun of It

Life sneaks little exercises in on you every day. You automatically do a sit-up when you get out of bed, toe touches every time you bend over to pick something up. Reaching for objects is mild stretching, and going up and down stairs gives your thighs and calves a mini workout!

Contrary to popular belief, fitness is fun! There are so many types of sports and forms of enjoyable exercise that becoming fit can always be exciting. Yes, it can be hard work, but the rewards of a healthy, physically fit body are worth every drop of glistening sweat.

When I say "fitness" I am not talking about just losing weight. Being physically fit has little to do with your actual body weight. To be fit means to have lean, long muscles that are working to their full capacity in providing you with strength, energy, calorie consumption, flexibility, stamina, and all-around top-notch health. Exercise helps in weight loss, but more important, exercise is for physical fitness.

Many high schools have dropped physical education as a required class. This makes lots of girls happy because it saves them the hassle of changing clothes and getting sweaty in the middle of the day. But in the long run their bodies pay a great price.

"I get plenty of exercise because I'm always busy," you may say. But you can't fool your body. It knows the difference between busy work and true exercise. Busy work basically wears you out. It burns a few extra calories along the way, but it isn't what we mean when we talk about real exercise.

We are going to talk about two kinds of exercise: aerobic and nonaerobic. Each kind achieves different results. Aerobic exercise involves not only many of your body's muscles but also your heart and lungs. Nonaerobic exercise firms and tones specific muscles for strength, coordination, and stamina. Most of us want a combination of the two for a complete exercise program.

I suggest that, before you begin an exercise program, you have a physical exam by your doctor so that you can eliminate any potential problems which exercise may complicate.

Aerobic Exercise

Aerobic means "air" or "oxygen." This is the kind of exercise you need to strengthen your heart and lungs, and to attack excess fat. We all carry a layer of fat between our skin and muscles. A woman's body is normally about 19 percent fat. Much more than that, and the fat will store up around our body, forming little rolls on our tummy and soft "saddlebags" on our hips that seem impossible to get rid of. Too much fat changes our shape and causes us to feel sluggish and apathetic. However, the goal is not to get rid of all body fat but to keep it at a minimum.

Carrying around excess fat does not necessarily mean that you are overweight. *Overfat* and *overweight* are not the same. You may be five feet, seven inches tall and weigh a mere 110 pounds. That certainly is not overweight. However, if you are proportionally more fat than you are muscle, you could very well be overfat.

Many thin girls think exercise is only for those who are plump. They think they don't need it. Not true. Everybody needs regular exercise. Also, proper exercise can actually help thin girls gain a little weight.

For an exercise to be aerobic, it must be performed for at least 12 to 15 minutes—*nonstop!* If you quit in the middle of your exercising, whether it's to get a drink or answer the telephone, your heart rate will drop and the aerobic effect is lessened. Your goal is to keep your heart working continuously at its training rate: 80 percent of its maximum working rate. You can test your heart rate during your exercise period by checking your pulse. Place your fingers, not your thumb, on your wrist or on the side of your neck. Count the number of beats in six seconds. Multiply that number by 10. You may need to get a watch with a second hand to do this efficiently. For teens, the average heart rate is between 160 and 180 beats per minute. This is your *training rate,* not your maximum rate.

Yes, I know you can get your heartbeat over 180 beats per minute, but don't! Overworking your heart will detract from your fitness goals. If your heart rate is high, simply slow down your exercise. Your body will be your guide. Obviously, if you can hardly breathe or are in overwhelming pain—*slow down!*

Speaking of breathing, *do* breathe while you exercise. Keep your breaths strong and deep. Concentrate on inhaling and exhaling. Take it in and blow it out!

As your body adjusts to your new amount of physical activity, you can

TOTAL FITNESS

work a little harder. If you have not been on an exercise program in a while, you may need to begin with only a fast walk or simple heel lifts. This may be enough to get your heart to its training rate. Always let your heart rate be your guide.

Following is a rundown on aerobic exercises. Remember, these exercises are aerobic because you do them without stopping! These exercises need to be done for varying lengths of time. Some are more strenuous than others. The times suggested are for those of you who are just starting an exercise program. Increase your time as you improve.

Walking

Fast walking, power walking, or as Weight Watchers call it, "pep stepping," is both fun and easy. Walking requires only a good pair of jogging shoes. It really is the best way to begin an aerobic exercise program—especially if you have not exercised in a long time or are overweight. Many doctors believe walking is the safest form of exercise for women. It works your heart and muscles without injuring your ankles, knees, or female organs. Some forms of aerobics jolt the body too much. Check your pulse to be sure you are walking fast enough. Don't be afraid to swing your arms while you walk! When you've worked up to it, add ankle weights. *Recommended walking time: 20 minutes.*

Jogging or Running

A decent pair of jogging shoes will get you started on this exercise. Jogging is probably the most popular form of aerobics. Always begin by stretching your ankles, calves, and thigh muscles. If you wear high heels very often, you especially need to stretch the backs of your ankles and your calf area. Begin jogging slowly and build speed after several weeks. If it hurts, stop! Overdoing it will leave you with shinsplints, strained muscles, and sore heels. Jogging on grass rather than hard pavement is easier on your body.

I used to jog too fast and could only last about fifteen minutes. My husband, Bill, an avid jogger, had to retrain me. I would be out of breath and ready for a jar of Gatorade before he was even warmed up!

Set a good, even pace, check your pulse, grab your shoes, and go jogging! *Recommended jogging time: 15 minutes.*

Swimming

Those of you on a high school swim team know what a complete workout you can get from swimming. Also, more of your muscles get in on the action when you choose to tackle the tide. Remember, though, for an exercise to be aerobic it must be done *nonstop*. Alternate the strokes you use—sidestroke, breaststroke, back swim, dog paddle. Keep it fun and keep it going. Your local YMCA, health club, city park pool, lake, or backyard pool are handy places to swim. *Recommended swimming time: 15 minutes.*

Skating

Roller and ice skating become aerobic when you do them long enough and hard enough to keep your heart at its training rate. It is difficult to find a place to skate where you are not body bumping a bunch of other skaters or

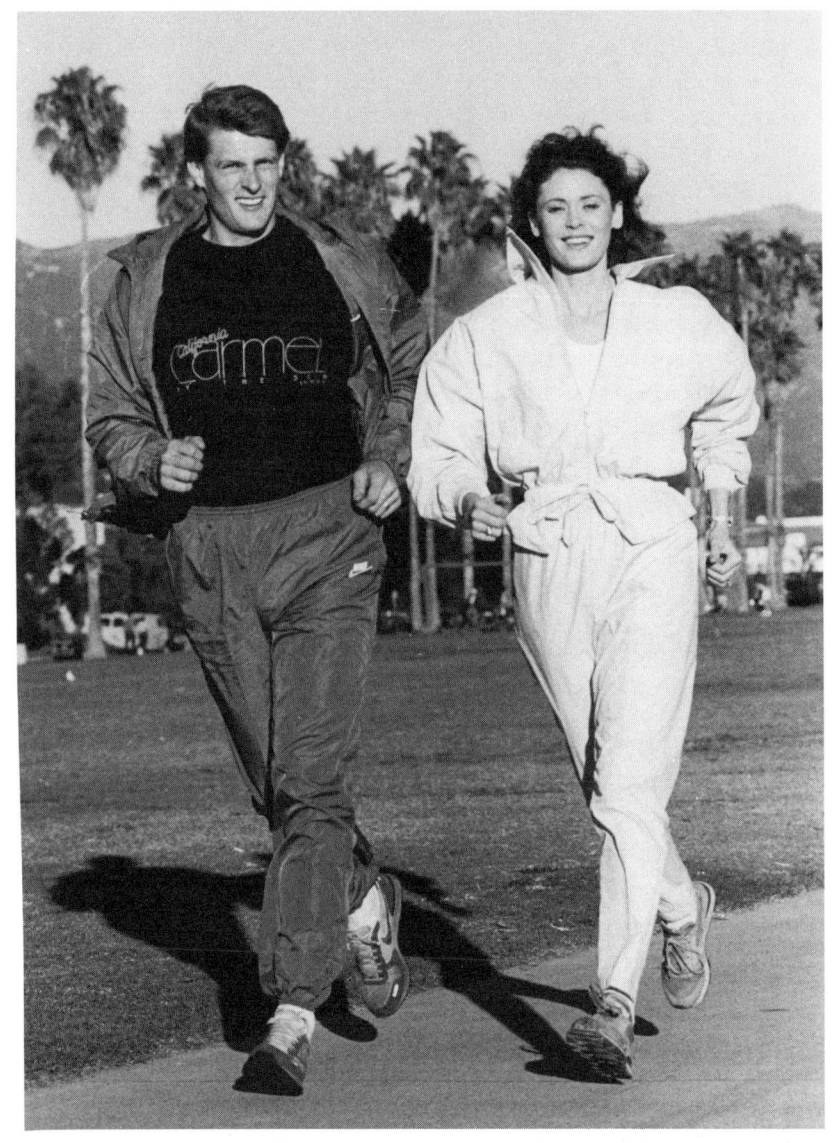

Pacing ourselves as Bill and I jog near the beach in beautiful Santa Barbara.

stopping for one reason or another. If you can find the right conditions, skating is great fun. *Recommended skating time: 20 minutes.*

Biking

Enjoy the country sights or city sights while you benefit your body by biking. Find a route with the fewest number of stop signs and traffic jams. Choose a sturdy bike with various speeds. This will help your heart remain at its training rate without forcing it to go higher every time you ride up a hill. Simply lower the speed on your bike to make the pedaling easier. *Important:* Wearing a helmet is a great safety precaution.

Indoor or stationary biking is just as good as outdoor. I enjoy putting on some music while I exercise. I even read while on my stationary bike. Just in case you are wondering, no, motor biking does not count here. It is not aerobic! *Recommended biking time: 20 minutes.*

Hiking

Hey, take a hike, kid! Mountain and bluff climbing can be quite aerobic as long as they are nonstop. Keep an eye on your pulse and the amount of time you climb. *Twenty minutes is a good minimum time for climbing.* Don't forget a canteen of cold water!

Cross-Country Skiing

Huh? It's true. This vigorous form of skiing can have great aerobic effects. No fair falling over in the snow after ten minutes, or trying to bribe someone behind you to push you along.

Obviously, if you live where it is warm year-round you'd better not set your heart on making cross-country skiing your number-one form of exercise. You do need snow! *Keep the skiing going at least 20 minutes.*

Dancing

Okay! Now we're talking! When I suggest aerobic dancing I do not mean learning all sorts of tricky steps that make you stop every two minutes to learn a new step. This start-and-stop learning is not aerobic. It will be aerobic when you have learned the routine and can repeat it for 18 minutes without stopping.

When I say *dancing* I am specifically referring to aerobic dance. Structured dancing for exercise is great. Dancing to attract attention or to get close to some guy is not so great. Dancing may be a controversial issue among some Christians because some forms of dancing can be very sexual or suggestive. I'm sure you know what I mean.

There are many Christian aerobic cassettes and videotapes available. In my opinion, aerobic dance is the most enjoyable form of exercise. I usually put on an Amy Grant or Michael W. Smith album. I make up my own routine as I go. Jumping jacks, can-can kicks, and jogging in place or around the room are wonderful fun. Check your pulse rate for six seconds, then multiply by ten. Keep your heart working within its training rate. Wear sneakers! Oh, one suggestion: You may want to do this craziness with your bedroom door shut! *Recommended dancing time: 15 to 20 minutes,* though you'll probably want to do it longer!

Jumping Rope

Secure your shoes, round up your rope, and start jumping! Choose a soft surface to save yourself from sore feet.

You will have to keep your mind active because jumping over and over can become challenging! This can be very strenuous, so *the recommended jumping time is 12 to 15 minutes.*

Machines

Rowing machines and treadmills are wonderful for aerobic effects. However, most of us do not have these fine pieces of equipment in our living rooms. You might have to join a health club to take advantage of these machines.

Aerobic Tips

1. Keep your exercises varied so you don't get into an exercise rut. Alternate your aerobic program. Be creative with your workout by choosing a couple of different exercises each week. Always remember to check your pulse rate several times to keep your heart within the recommended training rate. But wait—before you start, you must warm up your muscles!

2. To warm up your muscles, simply do a slower version of the aerobic exercise you plan to do that day. For example, if jogging is on your agenda for today, begin with a fast walk for 2 to 4 minutes. This allows your muscles to stretch and get prepared for a more strenuous exercise. It also saves you from sore, cramped muscles. Start counting the recommended amount of time *after* you warm up.

3. Do the same when you finish the timed part of your aerobic exercises (oh, relief). Slow down the exercise so your heart rate and muscles can cool down. Your cool-down time of 2 to 4 minutes will prevent soreness. Well, not completely! Well-worked muscles will feel well worked! Two to 4 minutes of warm-up, 15 to 20 minutes of aerobic exercise, then 2 to 4 minutes of cool-down time—a total of 20 to 28 minutes of workout time. Surely you can work this much time into your daily schedule!

Mild daily aerobic exercise is ideal, but 3 to 4 times a week is more realistic. Can you find 20 to 30 minutes every other day to commit to a healthier body? Is it worth the time and effort? I hope you will answer yes!

4. Those of you who expect immediate results from your exercise efforts, just relax! Being out of shape or overweight did not happen overnight. Neither will a new figure. Also, don't think that working harder at your exercise will bring quicker results. It won't. Exercising longer or more often, however, will. Be consistent, be patient, and you'll be pleasantly surprised with the results.

5. Make exercise a way of life for you. Don't cut exercise corners. Ride your bike to school instead of taking the bus or car pooling—or maybe even walk. Tackle the steps instead of riding the escalator or elevator. Keep your body in tip-top shape and remember: *Fitness is fun!*

Nonaerobic Exercise

Nonaerobic exercises include weight lifting, calisthenics, isometrics, and isotonics. All of these are nonaerobic, spot-firming exercises. This type of exercise does little for fat deposits surrounding the muscle. Rather, it concentrates on forcing fat out of your muscles and on toning the muscles themselves.

These exercises work on one muscle at a time. For example, when you do a sit-up, you are primarily working your abdominal muscles; you are doing little for your upper arms. Likewise, side stretches may make your waist smaller because of the toned muscle, but your calves aren't getting a whole lot out of the experience.

Spot exercises are good not only for firming and reducing but also for warming your muscles before your aerobic exercise. Warming your muscles as an early-morning wake-up is a great idea, too!

The place where you carry excess weight is the first place you will want to attack! What we can see we go after!

Figure 4-1   Figure 4-2   Figure 4-3   Figure 4-4

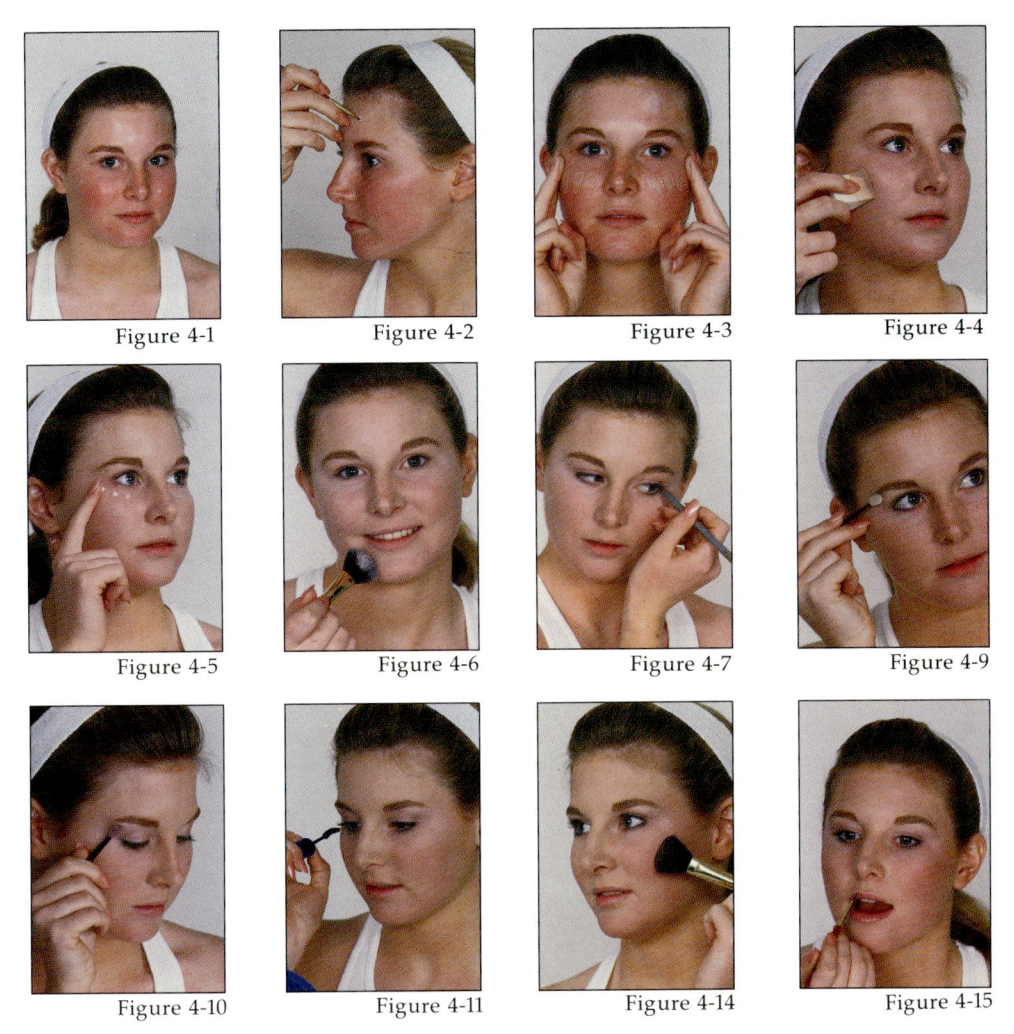

Figure 4-5   Figure 4-6   Figure 4-7   Figure 4-9

Figure 4-10   Figure 4-11   Figure 4-14   Figure 4-15

Row 1, Left to Right: Begin with clean, moisturized skin. Cover breakout with light cream before foundation or use additional foundation on breakout after initial foundation and powder. Rub foundation on first two fingers, press onto skin. Use makeup sponge to smooth and blend foundation. *Row 2, Left to Right:* Dot light cream under eye and extend toward hairline. Blend. Powder entire face. Apply liner, connecting top and bottom line at outer corner. Smudge. Apply highlighter on lid from lashes to eyebrow. *Row 3, Left to Right:* Apply medium-toned shadow on outer three-quarters of eyelid and into crease. Add darker shade if desired. Blend. Tip ends of lashes with mascara. Coat them again, using the full wand, twirling it as you go. Control blush, beginning with light strokes. Stay on cheekbone. Add a touch of shimmering gloss over lipstick, or use colored gloss. *Row 4, Left to Right:* Pretty as a picture. Matching shadow, blush, lip, and nail colors gives a more natural, complete look.

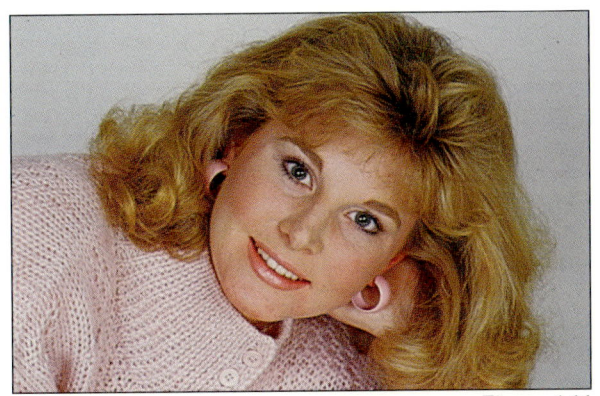

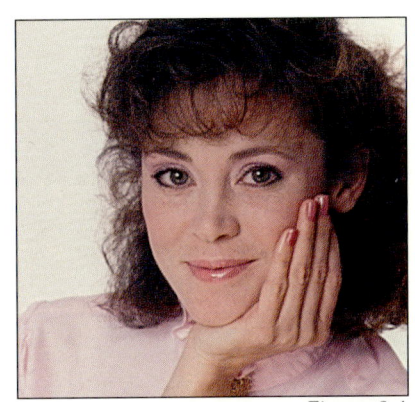

Figure 4-16   Figure 8-4

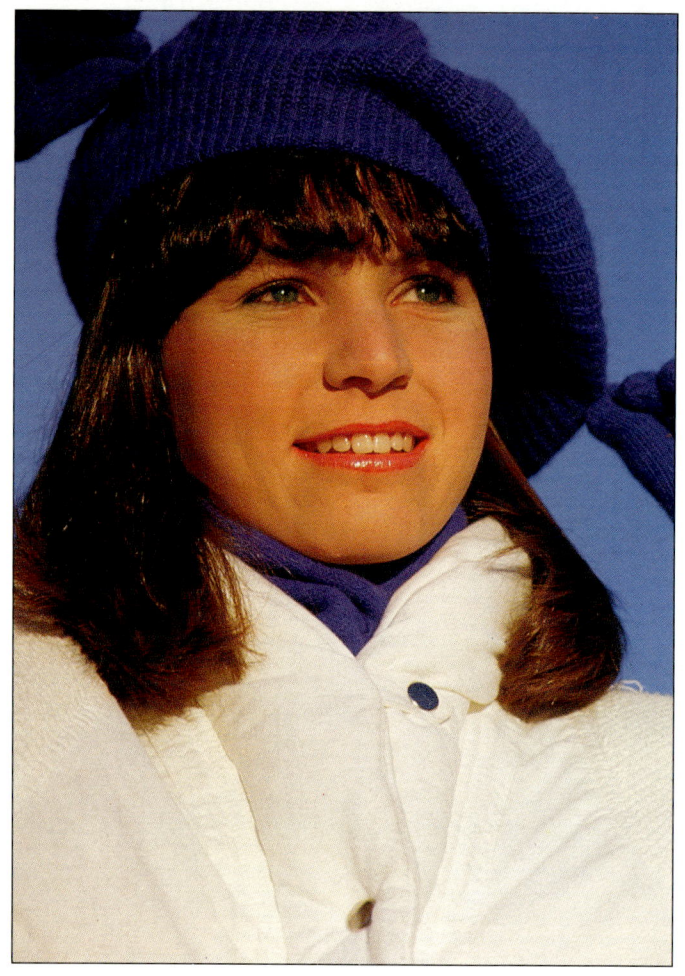

Winter

Amy's snowy white skin glows softly in the sun. Her near-black hair and gray-green eyes make her a perfect Winter.

Figure 9-2

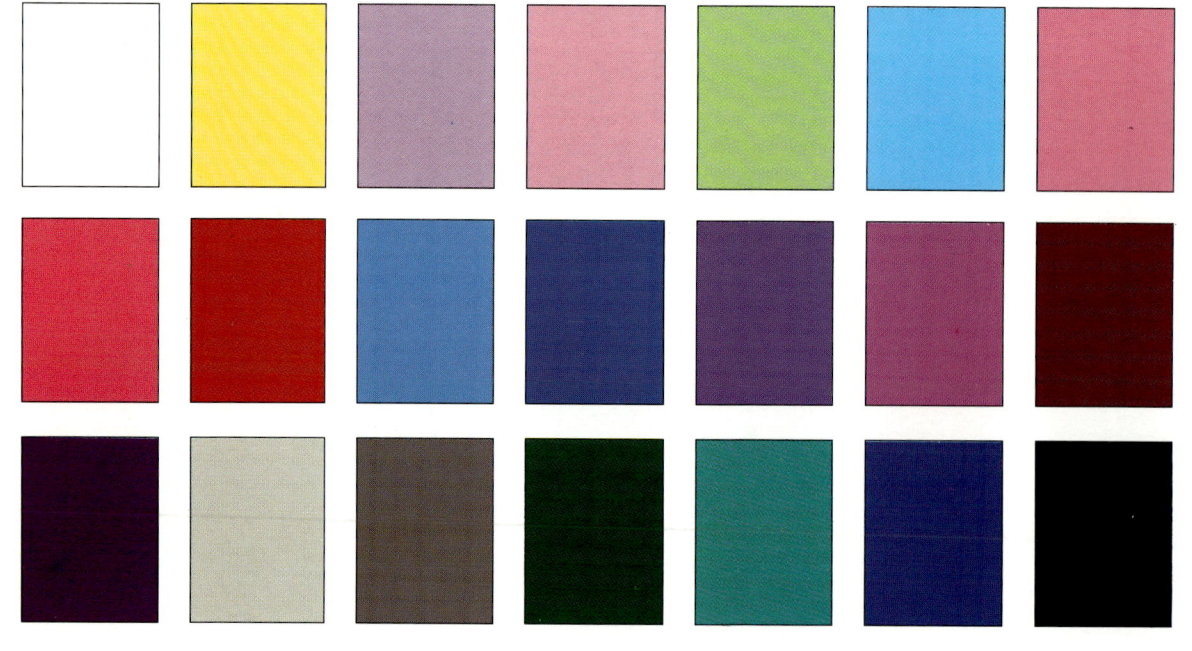

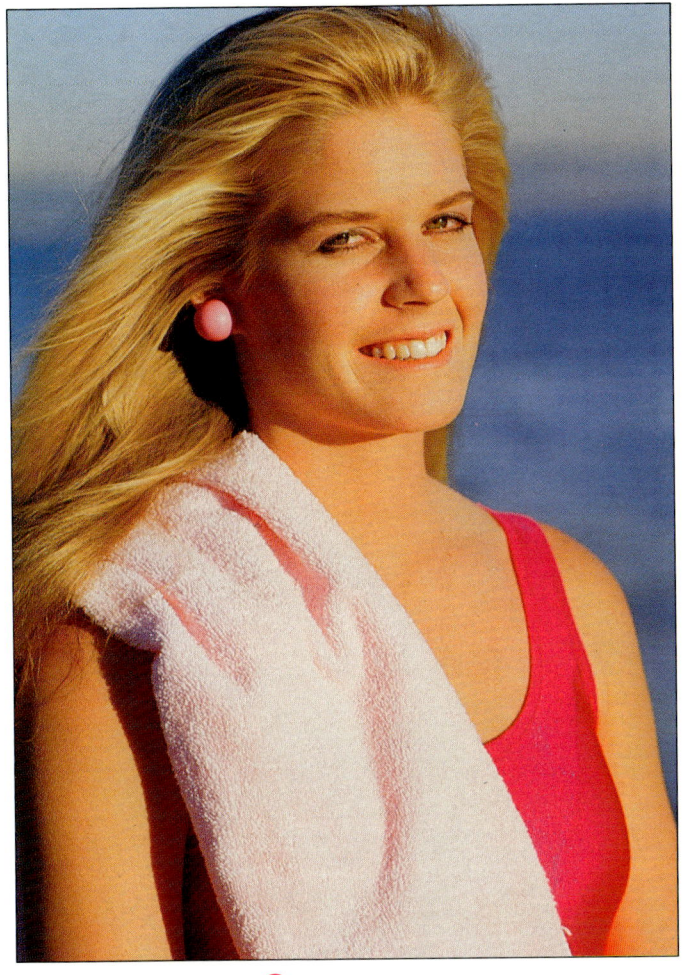

Summer

Kara has the gray-blue eyes, white-blonde hair, and fair skin tone typical of a Summer.

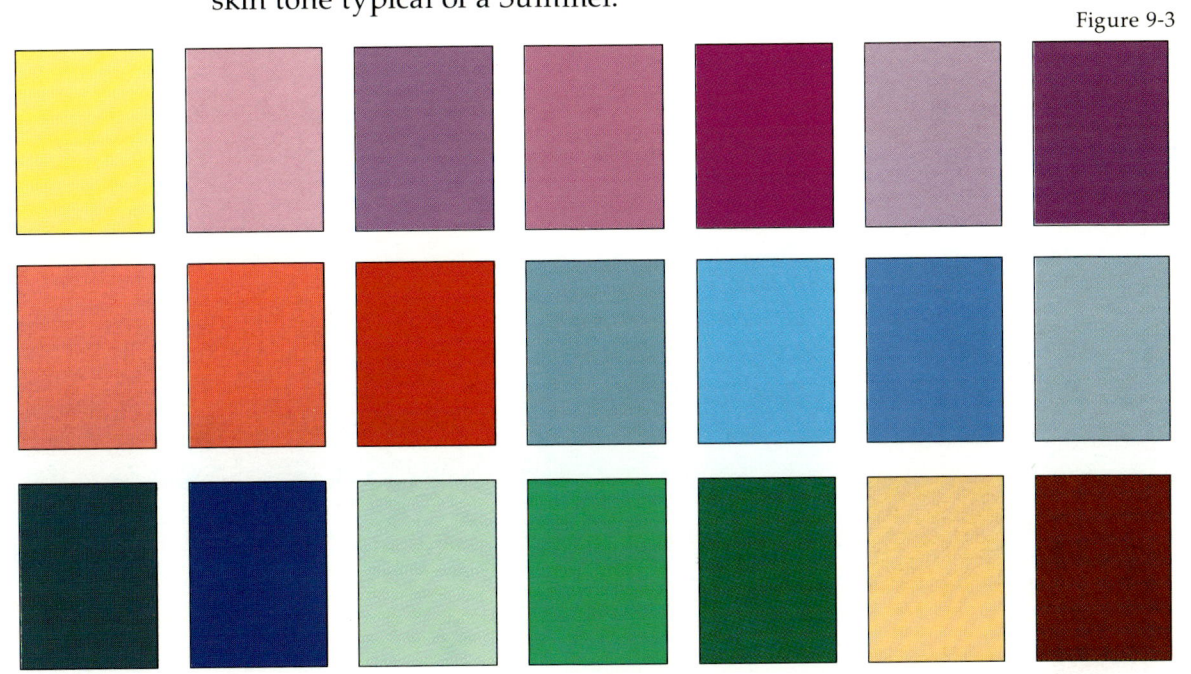

Figure 9-3

Spring

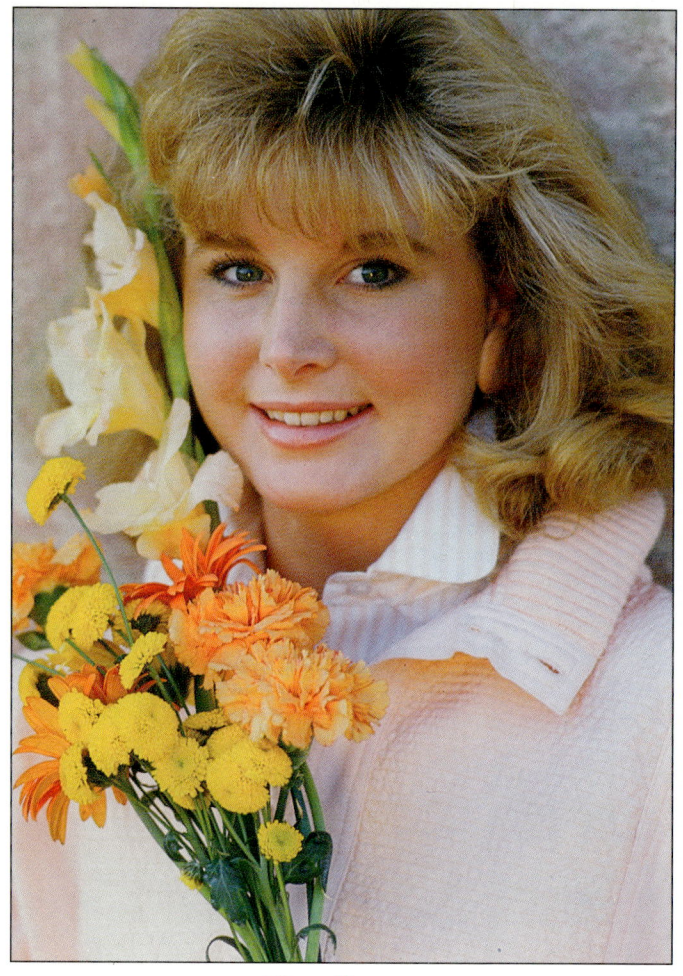

Creamy ivory skin, golden-blonde hair, and blue-green eyes put Kim right into the Spring season.

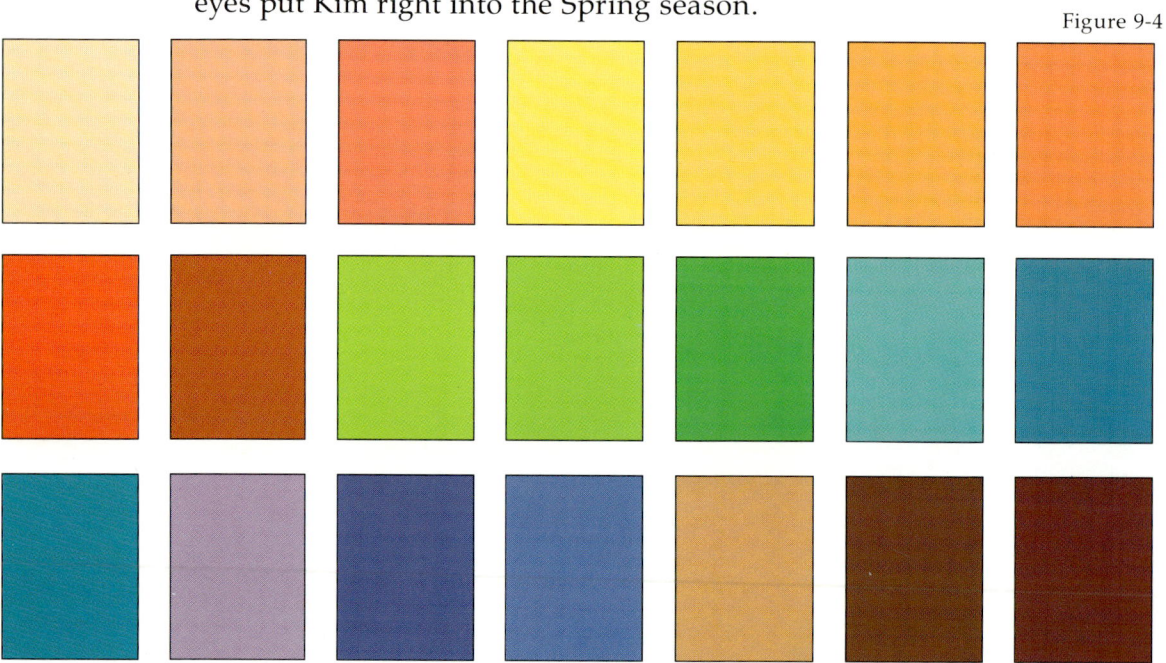

Figure 9-4

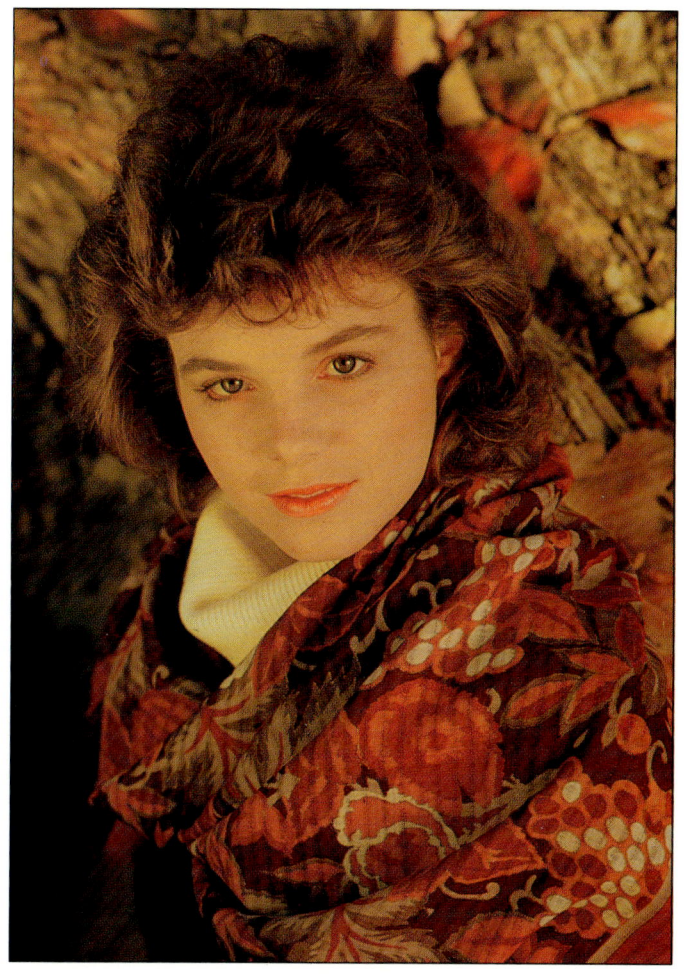

Autumn

Nicole has auburn hair, warm beige skin, and brown eyes
—all the beautiful shades of Autumn.

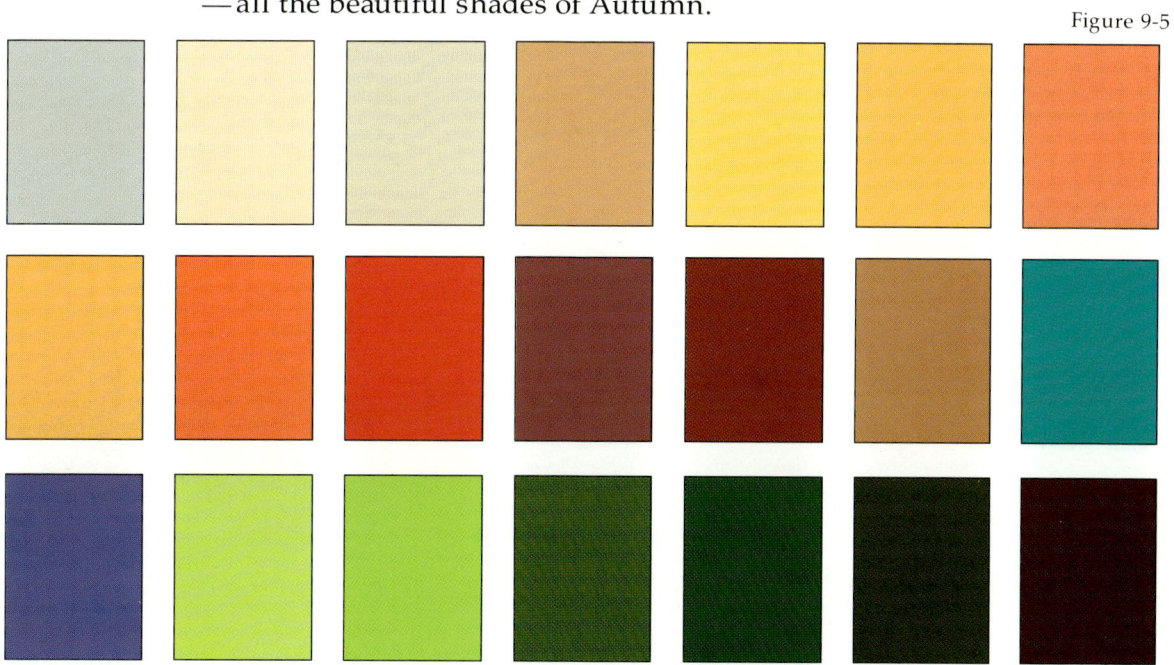

Figure 9-5

Basic Color Wheel
Figure 9-7

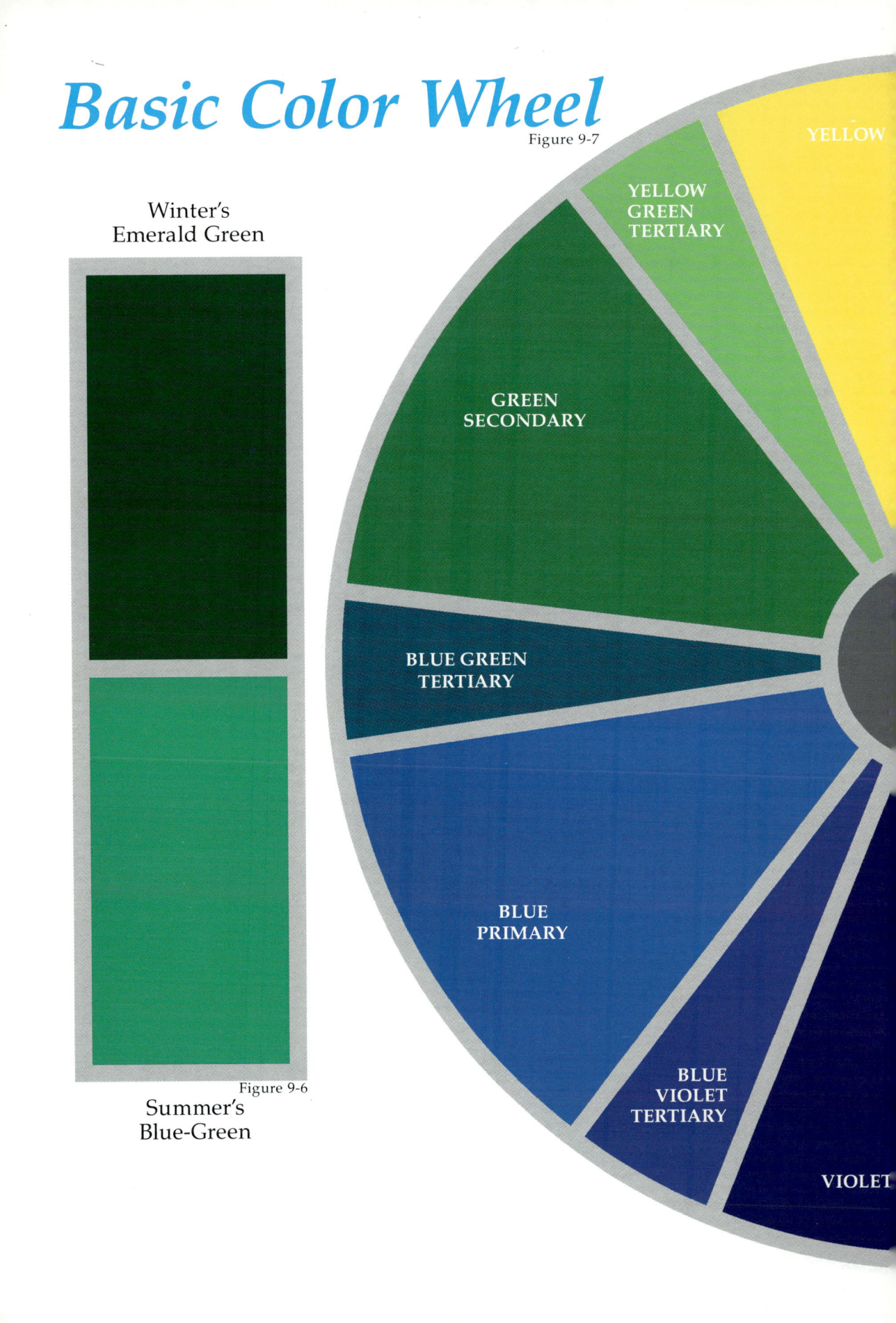

Winter's
Emerald Green

Figure 9-6
Summer's
Blue-Green

YELLOW

YELLOW GREEN
TERTIARY

GREEN
SECONDARY

BLUE GREEN
TERTIARY

BLUE
PRIMARY

BLUE
VIOLET
TERTIARY

VIOLET

PRIMARY

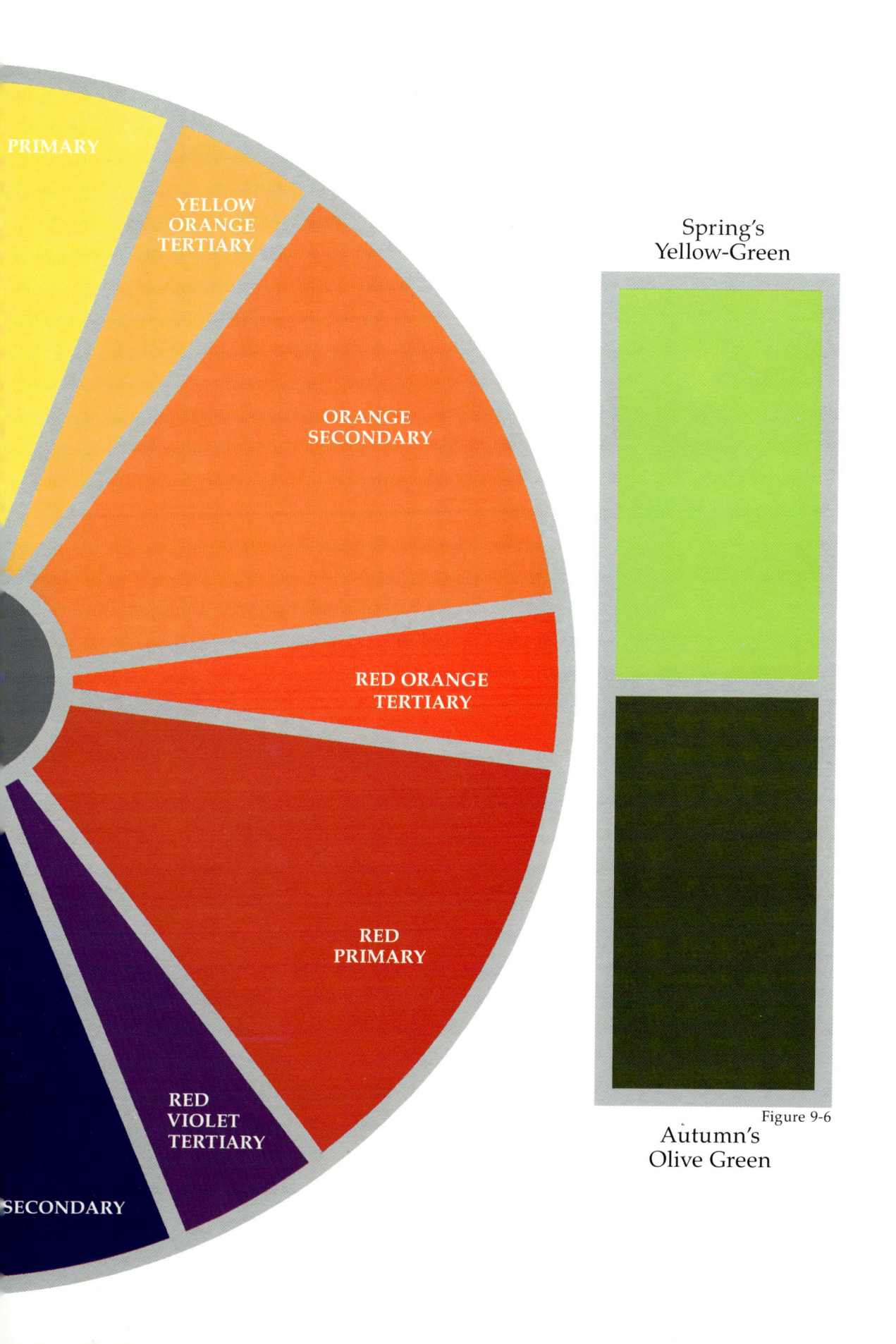

YELLOW
ORANGE
TERTIARY

ORANGE
SECONDARY

RED ORANGE
TERTIARY

RED
PRIMARY

RED
VIOLET
TERTIARY

SECONDARY

Spring's
Yellow-Green

Autumn's
Olive Green

Figure 9-6

Figure 9-8
Analogous Color Scheme

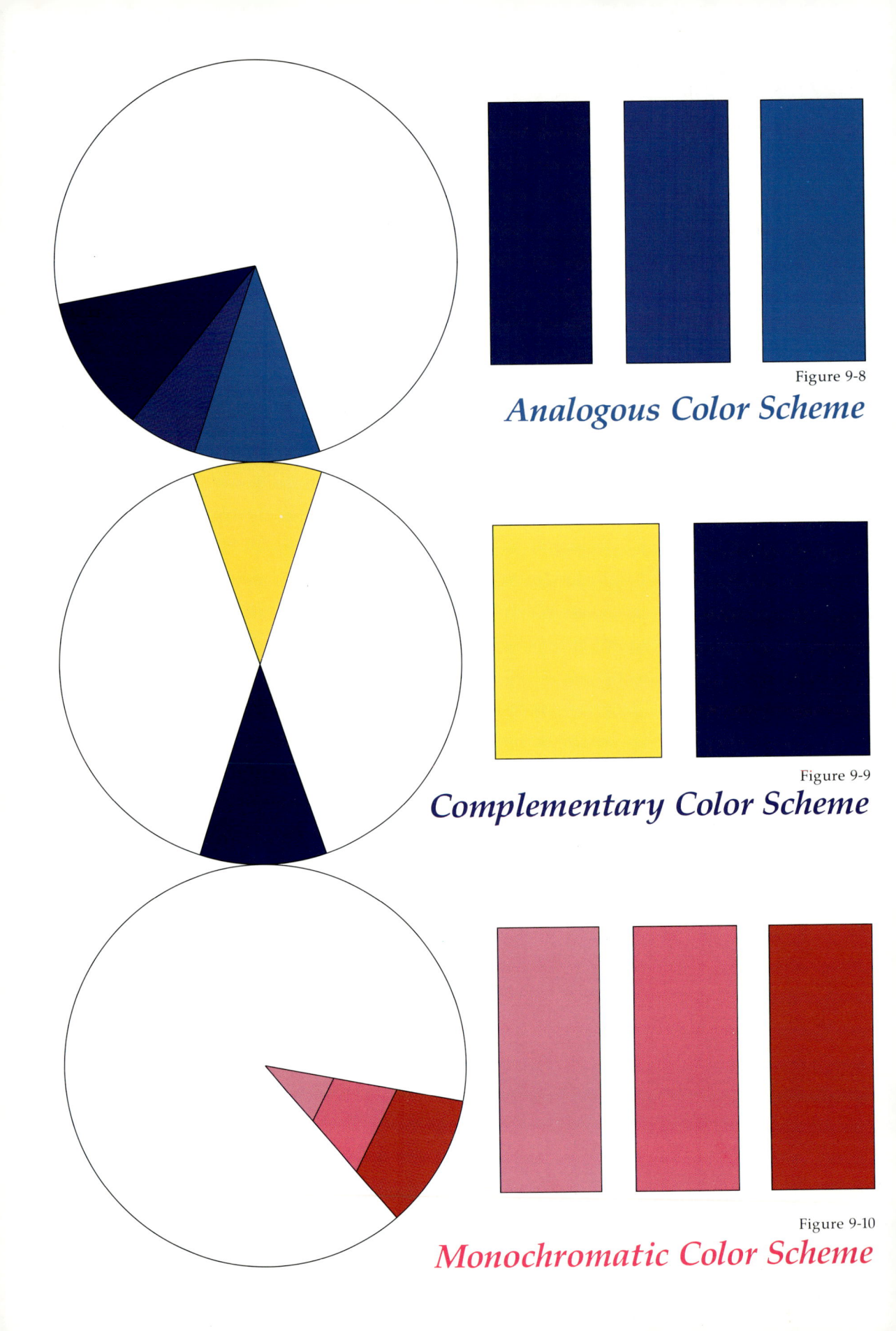

Figure 9-9
Complementary Color Scheme

Figure 9-10
Monochromatic Color Scheme

Just don't forget that all of your muscles need exercise to stay toned—whether they look toned or not.

Lifting weights has become extremely popular with women. Adding ankle and wrist weights to the exercises I have included is a great way to begin a light weight-lifting program. Weights are to be used every other day. The results will be well-defined muscle shape and increased muscle mass. No, you won't start looking like a guy if you lift weights. The female physique is different from the male physique. Nice muscle tone with a touch of definition looks feminine and appealing.

For a real change of pace, try doing spot exercises in the water. Swimnastics, aquacise, waterobics—all names for exercising in the H_2O. I don't always have a pool available to me, but when I was modeling I was a member of the New York Health & Racquet Club. It had a great pool and I took full advantage of the water exercise classes. It looks effortless, but the pressure of the water makes the exercises harder than normal. I always seem to be able to work out longer in the water than
out of it. You can even jog in the water. Your heart rate goes up but your body feels cool from the refreshing splash surrounding you. Give it a try.

Again, exercise pays off eventually. Don't be discouraged if your mirror's reflection is not what you desire for your body shape. Hard work and dedication can help you sculpt a new look.

Remember, when I say *body shape* I am talking about areas of excess weight that have changed your basic figure. Your basic figure is determined by your bone structure. Exercise cannot change your God-given bone structure. Accept what you cannot change as part of the unique you.

My lower hip is wider than the top of my hip. I can do 505 leg lifts, 750 hip rolls, and 1001 back leg kicks a day, and my hip structure will still be the same. Maybe you have a similar situation. It is all part of loving ourselves just the way God made us!

Following is a complete program for working out each part of your body. Always begin by slowly stretching your muscles. Do not bounce or force your muscles to stretch beyond the tension point. As you improve, you will see flexibility increase.

I suggest repeating each exercise 10 times. As you become familiar with the workout and your body adjusts to exercising, increase this to 15, then up to 20. You may repeat the exercise 20 times in a row, or alternate it by doing 2 sets of 10. For example, do 10 sit-ups, then 10 hip rolls, then 10 sit-ups, then 10 hip rolls. If performing all of these exercises is too strenuous or time-consuming at the beginning, choose one exercise for each part of your body. And if it hurts too much, stop. Work yourself up to the entire set of exercises. Shall we begin?

Head and Neck Area

1. Start at the top with head rolls. Gently bend your chin toward your chest. Slowly roll your head to the right, looking over your right shoulder, then slowly roll your head forward and to the left, looking over your left shoulder. Repeat exercise for a total of 10 times.

2. Shoulder rolls. Lift your shoulders up toward your ears, then slowly roll them to the back, down, forward, and return to the uplifted position. Repeat 5 times, then reverse the direction, for a total of 10 times.

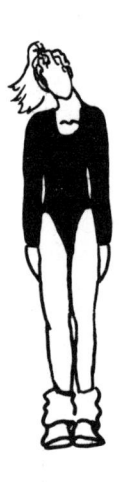

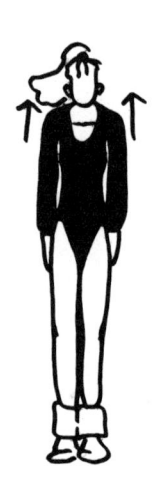

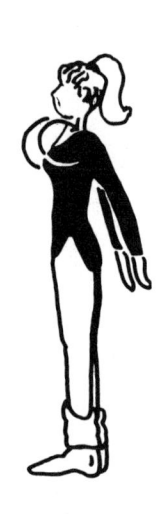

Arms

3. Hold your arms straight out to your sides at shoulder level, palms faceup. Bend your elbows so your fingers are touching the tops of your shoulders. Straighten your arms. Repeat 15 times.

4. The big windup—better known as arm circles! Start with your arms straight out at shoulder level. Begin making small circles, rotating your arms forward. Enlarge the circles as you go. Repeat, rotating in the opposite direction. Ten circles each way is good for starters on this exercise!

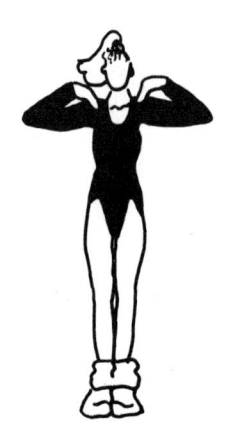

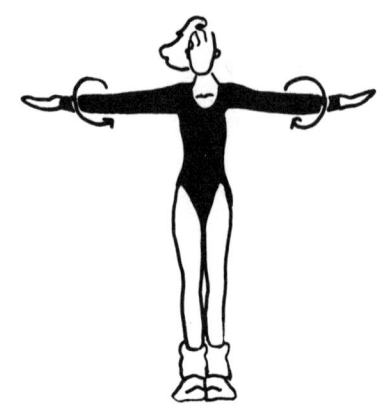

Upper Back and Chest Area

5. While standing, place your forearms on top of each other, making a big square. Be sure your arms are shoulder level. You'll look like an Indian chief! Now pull your arms back as far as you can. Hold for one second, then return to starting position. Repeat 10 times.

6. With your arms straight out and up in front of you, press your palms together with much resistance. Hold to the count of 3, then release. Repeat. This is great for your upper arms and chest. To make this exercise effective for the backs of your arms, cross your forearms and turn your hands, placing your palms together. Press and release. Start with 10 and build up!

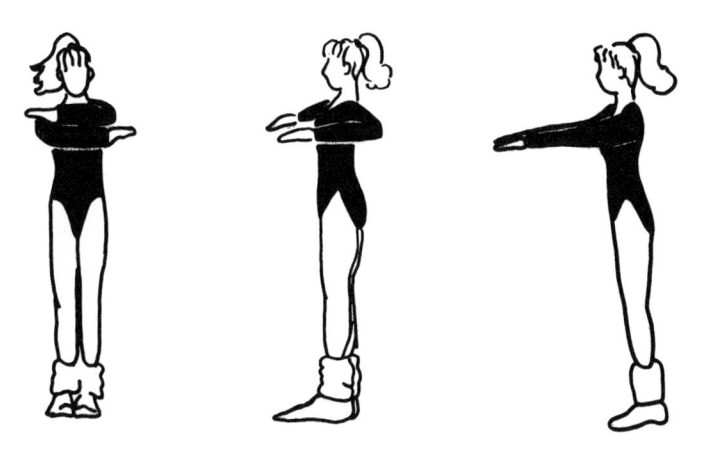

7. Down on the floor for this one! Start facedown with your arms straight out in front of you. Now lift your arms, head, and shoulders off the floor. Hold and relax. Do not strain your lower back. The pull should be in the upper-body area. Begin with 5, slowly working up to 12.

8. While you are on the floor and facedown, clasp your hands together behind you and pull, lifting your head and upper body. Hold and relax. Repeat 10 times. These last two exercises are great for improving your posture!

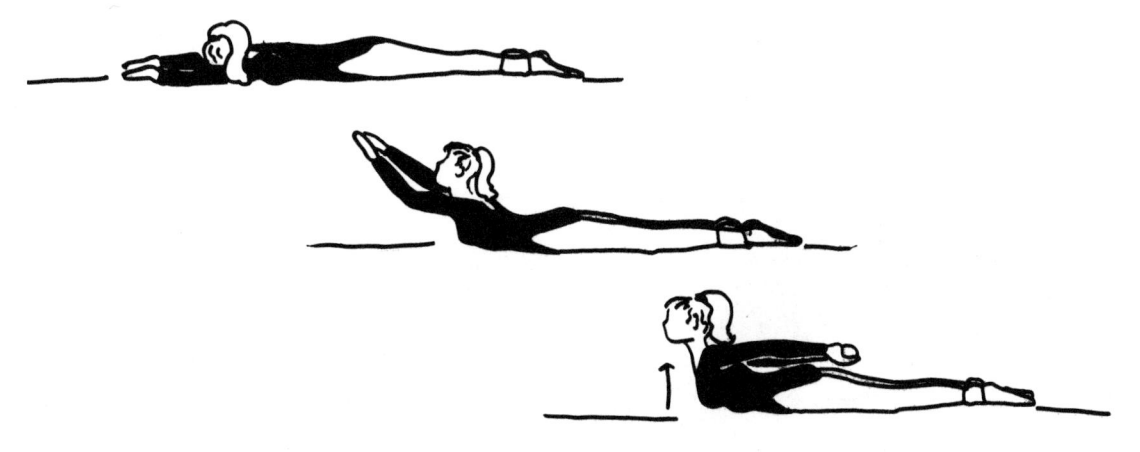

Waist Away

9. A good waist trimmer will work on muscles down your sides and mid-area. Start with a full stretch, reaching for the sky, as high as you can. Now, with your hands over your head, reach out to the right for 10 counts, then to the left for 10 counts. Really stretch. Feel the pull in your waist?

10. Next, bend forward at your waist with your arms out and slightly bent at your elbows. Keep feet apart. Twist from side to side, moving your head with your upper body. Repeat 10 times.

11. Now straighten up, but flex your knees. Tighten your buttocks, arms up and elbows bent. Twist again from side to side. Use control! Twist 10 times.

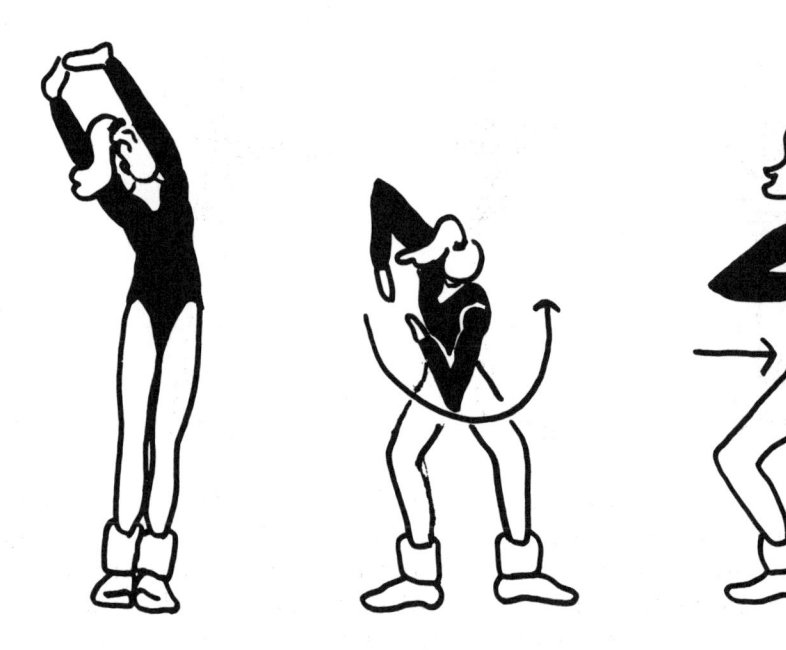

12. Sitting on the floor, prop yourself up with your arms. Keep left leg straight, right leg bent. Now cross your right knee over your left leg. Stretch your waist. Repeat 10 times, then change legs.

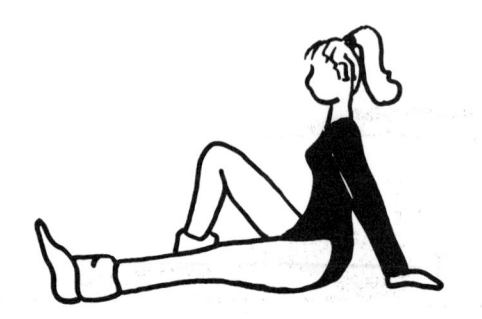

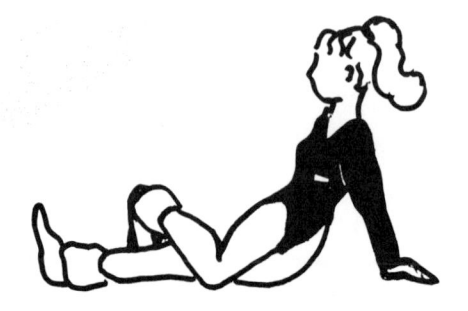

TOTAL FITNESS

Lower Back and Backs of Legs

13. Toe touches! Standing with your feet together, bend over slowly toward the floor. Do not bounce, just hang there. Relax your lower back. Feel the stretch in the backs of your legs? Repeat 5 times.

14. Since you are already hanging there, grab hold of your ankles. Stretch. Now try walking 4 steps forward, then 4 steps backward. Don't fall over!

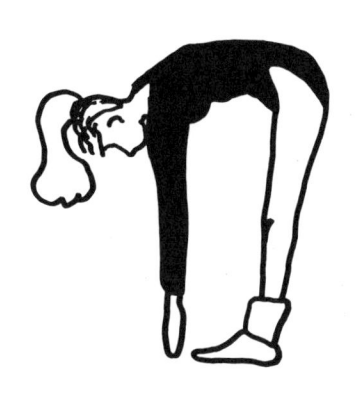

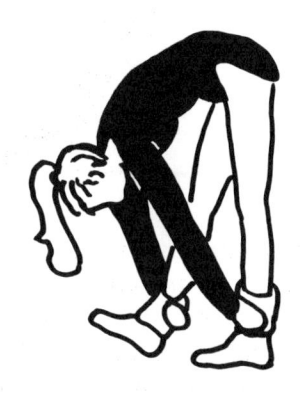

15. Now stand with your feet spread about 2 feet apart. Bend over, touching your left foot, then center, then right foot. Return to uplifted position. Repeat 10 times. For an extra challenge, try walking your hands out on the floor in front of you to stretch the backs of your legs and calves. Try keeping your heels on the floor.

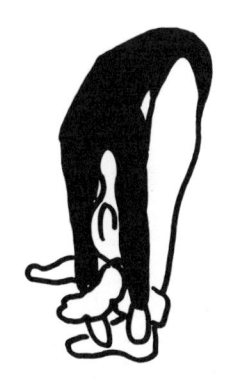

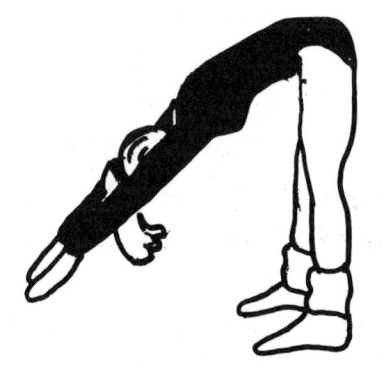

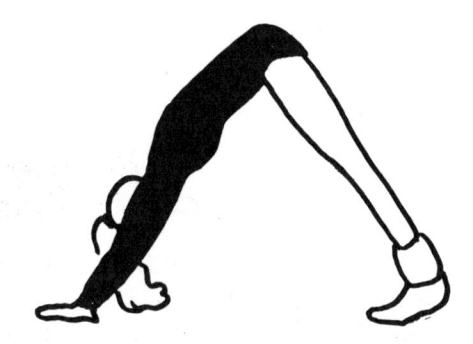

Abdomen

16. For your upper abdomen, lie flat on your back with your arms to your sides. Now lift your head and shoulders up off the floor about 10 inches. Hold, then relax, slowly lowering yourself to the original position. Repeat 5 times, adding 2 each week.

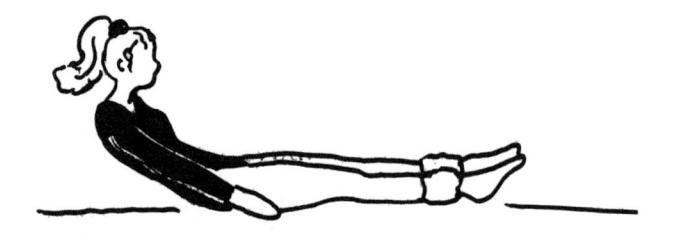

17. Lower abdomen next. Lie on your back with your hands under your buttocks for support to your lower back. Lift your legs off the floor 12 inches. Your knees should be slightly flexed. Slowly lower your legs to the floor. Oooh! Don't fret, these get easier as your muscles are toned! Begin with 5, working up to 10.

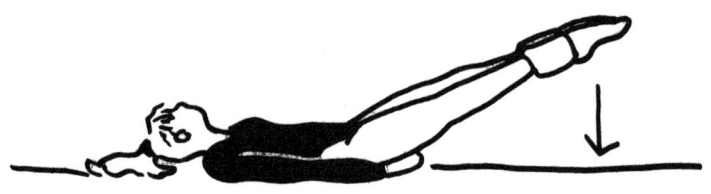

18. Try holding your legs 12 inches off the floor, then spread and cross, making a scissors motion. Repeat 10 times, then relax.

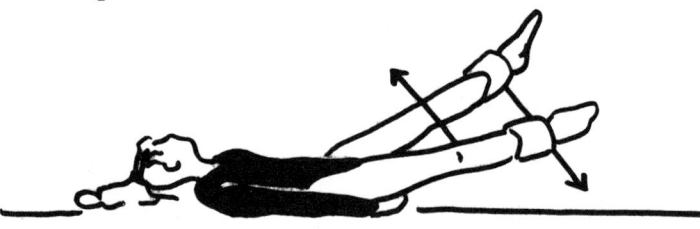

19. Oh, no. I wouldn't dare forget sit-ups. There are many ways to do these, but this one is good for beginners. Lie on your back, hands behind your head. At the same time, lift your head to your chest and your left knee to your right elbow. Touch and relax. Now the right knee to the left elbow. Ten is okay to start with. Work up to 50. Here is a good example of being able to make your muscle hard as a rock but still have soft tissue on top! Aerobic exercise needs to be combined with these spot exercises!

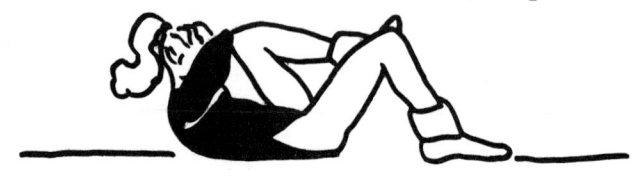

Inner Thigh

20. Standing with your feet 3 to 4 feet apart, knees bent, and hands on the floor, lunge toward the left, then to the right. Begin slowly in order to stretch, not pull, your muscles. Lunge 10 times to each side.

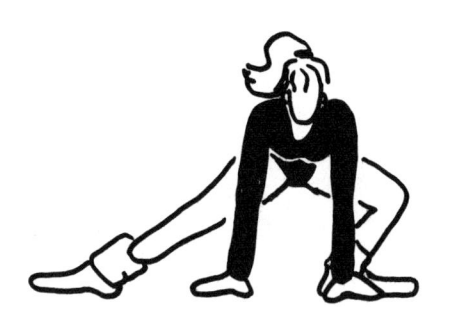

21. Sitting with your legs as far apart as you can, reach to the left, center, right, and up. Try this with your toes pointed, then flexed. Repeat 10 times.

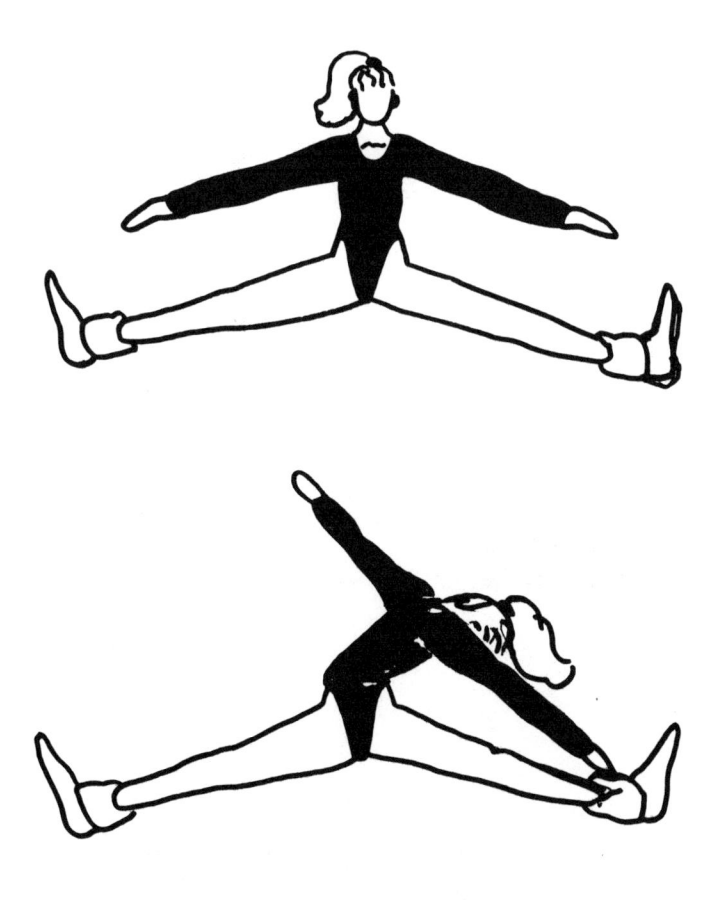

22. On your side, do 10 leg lifts. Stretch that inner thigh muscle. Now roll your hip slightly forward. Point your toe down toward the floor and do 10 more lifts. This position works on your outer thigh and the back of your leg.

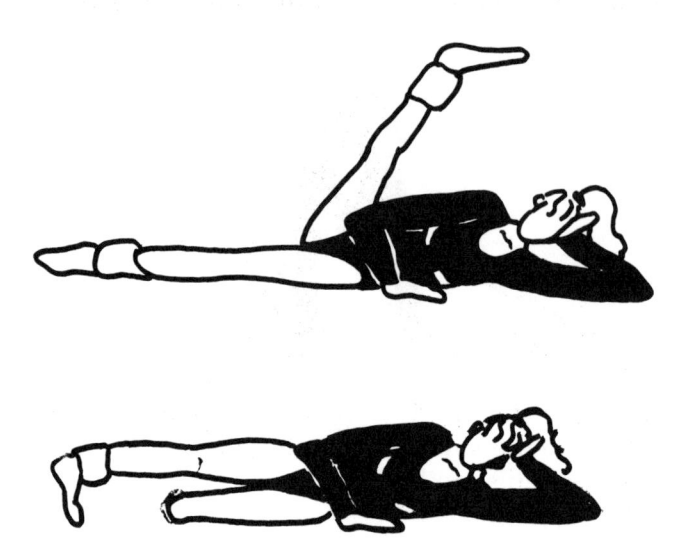

23. Begin on your back with your legs straight up from your hips. Cross them, stretching the outer thigh, then open them, stretching the inner thigh. Support your lower back by placing your hands under your buttocks. Repeat 10 times.

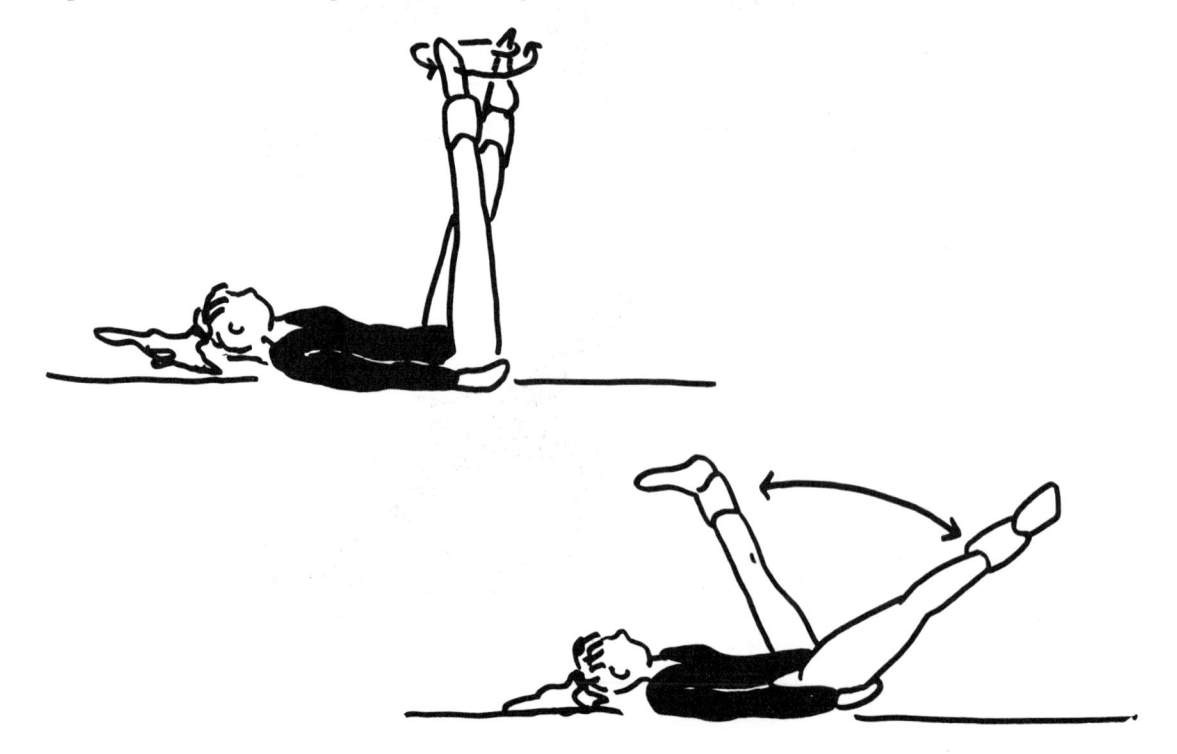

TOTAL FITNESS

24. This one leaves you feeling all twisted up! Ready? Lying on your left side, support yourself with your left forearm. Your left leg is straight, your right leg is bent, and your right foot is in front of your left knee. Hold your right ankle with your right hand. Now lift your left leg. Lower slowly. Repeat 10 times and change sides.

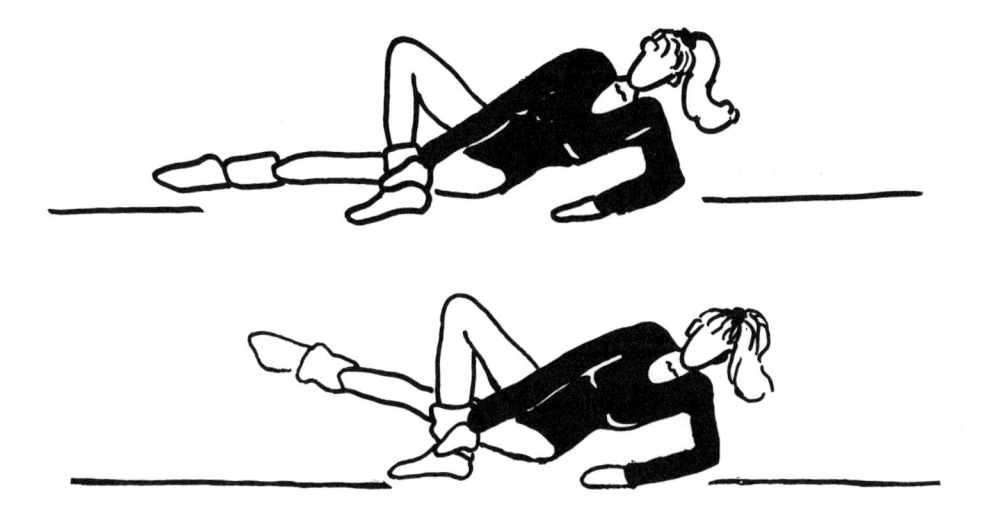

25. Your inner and outer thighs will love this! Stay on your side, one leg on top of the other. Lift them both this time. Smile, this is fun! Repeat 8 times, then change sides.

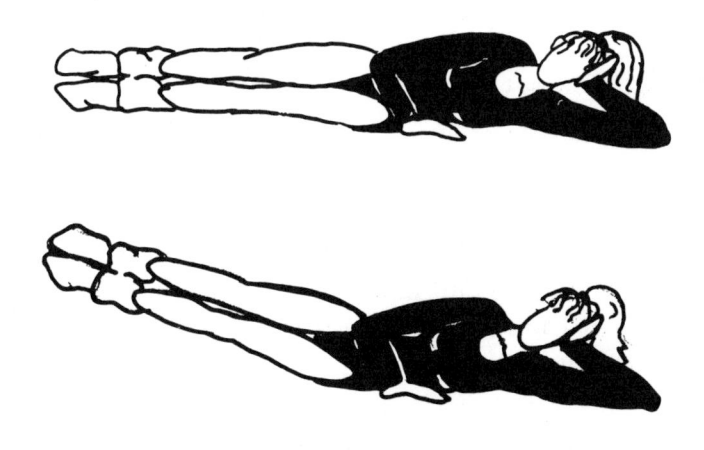

Outer Thigh

26. Bone up on your balance. Sit with both knees bent to the left. Balance on your right hip. Use your arms to keep you steady. Straighten your top leg out to the side, then back in. Repeat 10 times, then change sides.

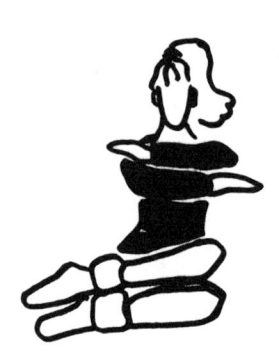

27. Fire hydrants! I've always dreaded this one, but it's very good. Therefore, you get to do it, too! Begin on all fours. Tuck by bringing your left knee to your chin. Now extend your leg back and up, head lifted. Repeat 10 times on each side.

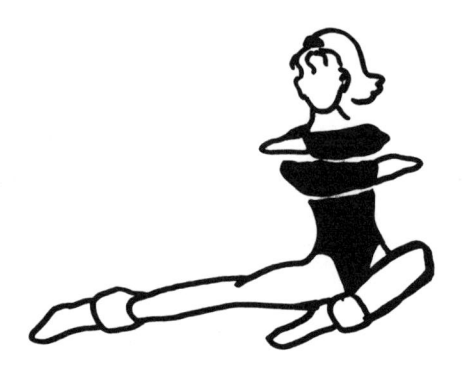

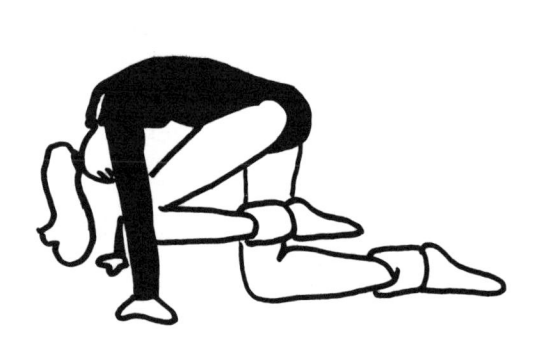

28. Now let's try it to the side. Instead of extending your leg back, lift it to the side, straighten it (point those toes), and return to starting position. Repeat 10 times, then change legs. When you get really good at these, add ankle weights.

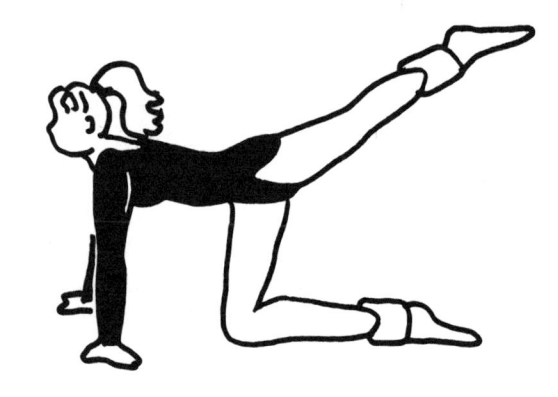

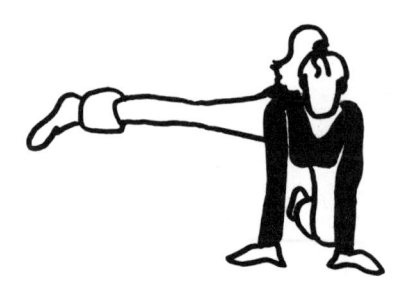

Hip Area

29. Now for your buns! This is the area that softens first. Unfortunately it is also probably the hardest to firm up. But the time spent is worth it. Okay, start by kneeling. Hold your arms straight out in front of you. Now slowly lean back, tightening your buttocks. Do not sit down. You will get a good stretch in your front thigh as you do this. Lift yourself back up and repeat 10 times.

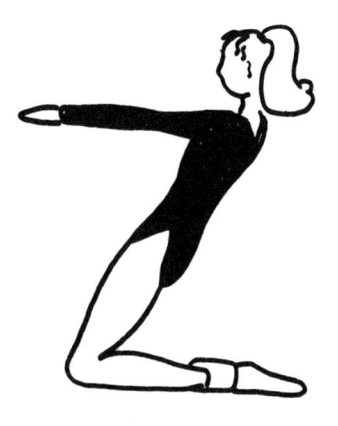

30. Lie facedown with your arms at your sides and your forehead on the floor. Lift both legs off the floor and do a quick set of 10 scissor kicks. Point those toes! Lower your legs, then repeat. You can place your hands under your hipbone to support your lower back.

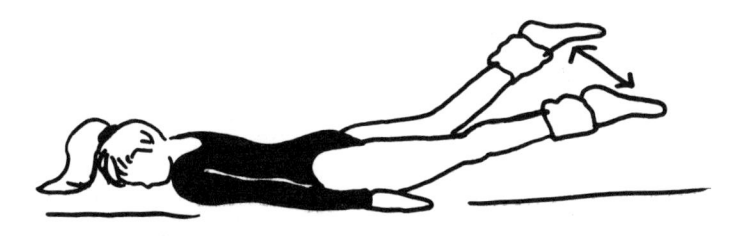

31. Next, roll over on your back, arms at your sides, feet about 12 inches apart and directly under your knees. Lift your hips to the ceiling, tightening your buttocks. Tighten and release. Lower your hips. Repeat 20 times.

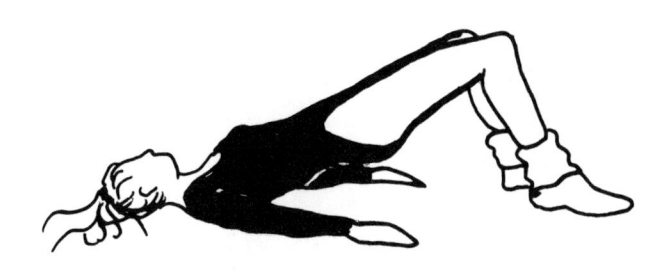

Calves and Shins

32. Last, but still very important, are your lower legs. Toned calves make for nice-looking legs. Hold on to the edge of a chair or the wall. Lift up on both sets of toes as high as you can. Now slowly lower your heels back down to the floor. Repeat 10 times.

33. For an extra challenge, balance the front half of your feet on the edge of a step. Lower yourself as far down as you can. Now, lift up as high as you can. You'll get a great stretch and great results! Repeat 10 times.

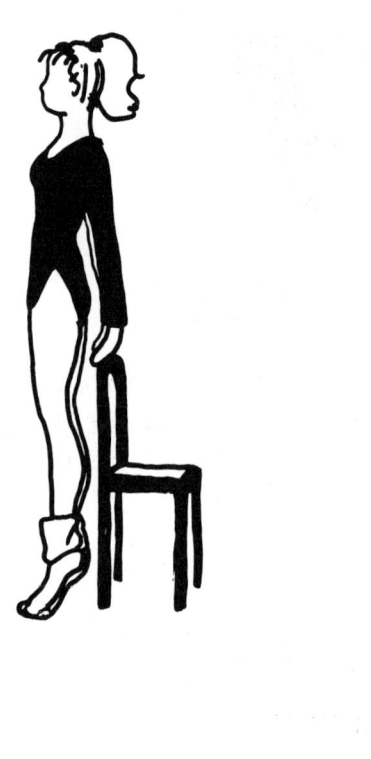

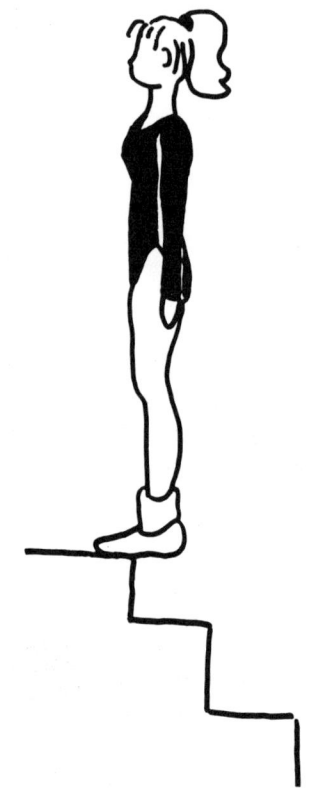

34. Shake out your whole body. Relax! Pat yourself on the back—you did it. Make yourself a chart listing each exercise and how many sets of 10 you do each time you exercise. Be serious and you will get serious results!

Exercise Chart

Make a chart similar to this one each month. Record the type of exercise you do and the amount of time you spend each day. Chart your results.

DATE	AEROBIC EXERCISES									SPOT EXERCISES			RESULTS
	Warm-up	Walk	Jog	Swim	Skate	Bike	Hike	Dance	Jump Rope	Cool Down	Spot Ex.	With Weights	Water Ex.	
Jan. 1	5 min.							24 min.		5 min.				Felt tired.
Jan. 2	2 min.									2 min.	15 min.	10 min.		Muscles felt worked!
Jan. 3														
Jan. 4														
Jan. 5														
Jan. 6														
Jan. 7														
Jan. 8														
Jan. 9														
Jan. 10														
Jan. 11														
Jan. 12														
Jan. 13														
Jan. 14														
Jan. 15														

Now you have no excuse for not getting started on an exercise program right away. You even have pictures to follow.

There are a few things I want you to understand about this exercise, toning, and weight-loss business.

First, results take time. The recommended amount of weight loss per week is one to two pounds. Eating right and exercising regularly will help your body find its most efficient operating level.

Second, measure your progress with a tape measure, not just a scale. Scales can be deceiving. Our body fluids fluctuate daily, and near menstruation time we retain water. The scale will show these changes, and it can be discouraging.

When you weigh yourself, do it in the morning with next to nothing on. Try to do it about the same time each day—only once or twice a week. Did you know that as your muscles get in shape, they will weigh more? It's true. Muscle tissue weighs more than fat tissue. So, you might even gain a bit. But as your exercising tones your muscles, the muscles themselves become longer, leaner, and slimmer. That means your weight may not change much, but you could lose inches off your thighs or waist because of the muscles changing shape. Exercise forces fat deposits out of your muscles so that they become more solid, longer, more feminine. Muscle tissue also burns more calories and gives you a healthier body. So, don't let the scale fool you.

Chart your progress with a tape measure. Measure yourself at the bust, midriff, waist, mid-hip (between four and five inches below your waist), lower hip (widest part, between eight and a half to ten inches below your waist), upper thigh, right above your knee, and your calf. Record the date. Check your measurements on a monthly basis. Set sensible goals.

Third, this sounds strange, but we usually gain weight in a specific order, then lose it in the reverse of that order. The first place we gain is the thighs, then hips, midriff, then arms. We lose in the opposite order. See if you can notice the changes.

The fourth tidbit to add to your exercise knowledge is that exercising might make you hungry—but it is only temporary. A few weeks into your

Measurement Chart

MEASUREMENTS	One Month Later	Two Months Later	Three Months Later	Four Months Later	Five Months Later	GOALS
Beginning Date BUST MIDRIFF WAIST MID-HIP LOWER HIP UPPER THIGH ABOVE KNEE CALF	_____ _____ _____ _____ _____ _____ _____ _____	_____ _____ _____ _____ _____ _____ _____ _____	_____ _____ _____ _____ _____ _____ _____ _____	_____ _____ _____ _____ _____ _____ _____ _____	_____ _____ _____ _____ _____ _____ _____ _____	_____ _____ _____ _____ _____ _____ _____ _____

program, you will find that you don't even want to eat when you are done! Well, not for an hour or so.

For those initial hunger pains, try drinking a glass of water or half a cup of juice. Don't run for the cookie jar! Always let your body cool down before you eat. It is said to be best to exercise before your meals rather than after. If you do work out after a meal, wait at least an hour before you start. Your blood is needed to assist your digestive system before it rushes off to your muscles.

Exercise Attire

When you work out, wear clothes you can move comfortably in. Clothes that are too tight may restrict your movement. If they are too loose, you'll be bothered with pushing up your sleeves or pulling up your sweat pants.

To keep your muscles warm, start out with several layers of workout clothes. Then you can shed them as your muscles warm up. Wearing a sweat shirt on top of a T-shirt or leotard will allow you to do this. Skip the sweat clothes during the hot summer months.

Tie your hair back away from your face so you don't have wisps of hair slashing you across the face while you are trying to concentrate. This helps keep the skin on your forehead from breaking out, too.

Speaking of skin, do not exercise with face makeup on! Mascara is okay, but no blush, foundation, or heavy creams. When your body becomes hot from the exercise, your facial pores open. If you have goop on your face, it will soak into your pores, resulting in clogged pores and possible breakout. Looking gorgeous comes *after* the exercising, not *during!* It always makes me cringe when I go to exercise class and I see women with their faces fully decked out. They may be helping their bodies but they are gagging their skin.

Always wash your face thoroughly before and after your workout. Follow with a touch of astringent and moisturizer.

My Exercise Autobiography

You don't have to be a jock to enjoy exercise. I am a perfect example of this fact. I like to exercise, but I'll never be called an athlete.

My early experiences with sports should have been an instant indication to me that I would never be an Olympic Gold Medalist. I was a very long baby and a frail toddler. As a kid, the big game in our neighborhood was kickball. Every night after dinner we all assembled in the vacant lot down the street. Each of us was eager and ready to pound the other team. All positions were equally important—first base, second base, and third, outfield, catcher; we were each skilled for our own special job. And what was my all-important position, you ask? Scorekeeper.

You know how most kids play games during recess in grade school? Well, I wasn't big on foursquare or hopscotch. I do, however, remember one day when I made unexpected contact with a softball.

My family had recently moved from a small town in Ohio to Madison, Wisconsin. It is never fun to be the new kid on the block. Not knowing many of my fellow classmates, I often found myself alone during recess. I know, I know, you think only the nerdie kids are alone during recess.

But that's not true! I was extremely shy. Okay—I'll get to the point. It was during morning recess. All the others were busy at play and I made the mistake of walking across the playground (minding my own business, of course). Suddenly, out of nowhere came a soaring softball that hit me right on the corner of my pointy-rimmed glasses! My glasses went flying across the playground. A tiny trickle of blood ran down my face. Feeling totally embarrassed and very silly, I picked up my glasses and with dignity I walked off the playground as if nothing had happened. I knew right then I would never be buddies with a softball!

Moving up into junior high gave me new hopes for my athletic career. I decided to be brave and go out for track with my friend Julie. Julie was and still is a jock through and through. In fact, she helped carry the official torch in the 1984 Olympics.

Surely there was nothing to running around a gravel track and jumping some funny-shaped things called hurdles.

On the first day I figured they were laying it on thick—just to weed out the wimps! Jumping jacks, stretches, sit-ups, laps—you name it, we did it. Lap after lap after lap. Coming up on what felt like my 105th time around that darn track, I realized the side door into the gym was open. Surely no one would notice I was gone. Closer, closer came the door, and in I darted. Whew! Relief at last. I thought I was safe until I heard our burly coach yell, "Andrea, get back out here."

Two days, yes sir, two days of track was all I could handle. My calves hurt so bad I could hardly walk up the stairs between classes. I was convinced people who ran track were crazy.

High school didn't bring many changes. In gym class I was nearly always chosen last for the basketball teams. Sad but true. I hated going to gym class!

As a junior, I decided to expand myself and take ballet lessons. Ballet seemed only mildly athletic, so my hopes of succeeding were high! My younger sister, Alisa, graciously joined me. The only openings at the Ballet Academy were in a class for nine- to twelve-year-olds. What the heck, we thought. So we joined.

All went fine until recital time. I had missed several lessons because I was performing in a musical at the high school. I didn't want to miss being in the recital because I knew I would probably never be in one again. So, even though I wasn't too sure of the routine, I did it.

You can guess what happened. There I was in the front row, in my powder-blue tutu, surrounded by little nine- through twelve-year-olds. They were so sweetly tiptoeing to the left while I was tiptoeing to the right! When the routine was over I ran out of the building and cried!

The highlight of my senior year was being crowned Madison's Junior Miss. I spent much time and effort preparing for the Wisconsin Junior Miss Pageant, to be held only a few months after winning my local title. There are five areas of competition in the Junior Miss program: scholastic achievement, poise and appearance, creative and performing arts (dressed as a hobo, I played "Mr. Bojangles" on my twelve-string guitar), judges' interview, and . . . physical fitness. I went to the state pageant ready for every area of competition and wanting to do my best. But please, why did they have to put push-ups in the physical fitness routine? I will never forget the night I performed the routine. Down on the floor in my swamp-water green outfit, I breezed through the leg lifts and sit-ups. Flipping over with grace and style, I began the ten push-ups. Oh, help, four, five, six, seven. My arms were weakening . . . eight . . . nine . . . that was it! I never went down for that tenth push-up! And can you believe I was laughing in front of the judges and everyone else! But in spite of my push-up mishap, I finished as second runner-up.

Even to this day, I avoid most sports. Just recently I was dragged into a volleyball game with the college group at our church. Terrific! Right away, the ball came straight at me! I locked my hands together and smashed that ball with my forearms. Straight up into the air it flew. I had my eyes closed as I always do when I see a volleyball flying toward me. And where did it land? *Bonk*—right on my head. Talk about ultimate embarrassment!

You don't have to be a star athlete to enjoy exercising. The suggestions I have given in this chapter are exercises anyone can do and benefit from. You will feel better, look better, and have more confidence by staying in shape. Physical and spiritual shape, that is!

Exercising Your Faith

To exercise your muscles means to use them. The result of continuous use is muscles that grow and develop. These developed muscles produce more for you than the ones you started with.

Faith works in a similar way. Faith means belief, trust, and confidence. When you act on your beliefs, your faith grows and develops. The more faith you have and the more mature your faith becomes, the greater strength you will have in your life, just as in your muscles!

Does faith start out big? Not usually. Jesus talks about faith beginning very small. He compares the size of faith to a mustard seed, which is tiny. As the mustard seed is given time and proper nourishment, it grows into a huge plant. Our faith might start small, but it has big potential. Jesus told His disciples that even with a small amount of faith, they could do great things. So can you.

Ever wonder how you can get that seed of faith to grow? I know of two ways. The first is to exercise it by using it, just as we exercise those underdeveloped muscles. But you never heard of faith push-ups—so how do you exercise faith? Very good question. Hebrews 11:1 describes faith as the evidence of something we hope for, the things we don't see yet. So, for example, let's say you know the Bible tells us that we have everlasting life the minute we accept Jesus as our Lord and Savior. Not everlasting physical life, but the real us, the spiritual part of us. We know that when our bodies die, the real us goes to heaven. Now, you've never seen heaven. Yet, with your little bit of faith you confirm that God's Word is true, and that will get you to heaven. When you express your faith you exercise it so that it grows. It's the same way for any Christian principle you believe in. (*Faith* and *Belief* are the same words.)

Another way to exercise faith is through prayer. God promises to answer prayers, so you stretch your faith expecting the answer to come. It might not be the answer you hoped for, but

God responds to your faith and to the promises in His Word.

Solid faith is based on the Word of God. In fact, Romans 10:17 tells us that faith first comes to us by hearing the Word of God. The more we hear and read the Bible, the more solid our faith or set of beliefs will become. So this is the second way we get more faith, by hearing God's Word and putting it into practice—or exercising it. To keep your faith in shape, believe God for things in your life. Expect Him to work in you and through you. Learn more about Christian faith from the Bible and, like that tiny mustard seed, your faith will blossom into a giant plant.

Stretch your faith! Give it a workout. What are you needing and wanting from God today? Ready? And one, and two, and three, and stretch!

TOTAL FITNESS

Project Page

1. Describe what it means to be physically fit. _____

2. What is the difference between overweight and overfat? _____

3. Define *aerobic* exercise. How does it differ from *nonaerobic* exercise? _____

4. Determine your heart rate during your exercise time by counting the number of heartbeats in 6 seconds. Multiply that number by 10. For safety reasons you should never exceed 180 beats per minute.

5. Using the chart on page 109, keep an exercise journal. Be specific and be consistent!

6. To exercise your faith, you must use it. What situation in your life is urging you to use your faith? Are you using your faith?

7. Expecting answers to your prayers is also a way to exercise your faith. Make a prayer list similar to this one. Be sure to write in the date of the prayer and the date God answers it!

DATE	PRAYER REQUESTS	DATE ANSWERED
	1.	
	2.	
	3.	
	4.	
	5.	

7 HAIR HAPPENINGS
Styles That Give You Style!

It blows out of place with even the slightest wind, goes limp in humid weather, curls opposite the way you planned, needs daily attention, and often steals more time than it is worth.

Hair. It sometimes has a mind of its own, creating styles we never dreamed of. Nevertheless, we have it and are better off with it than without it. Bald is not in these days!

Our hair is actually a great covering for our scalp and a real way to "top off" our appearance. The Bible says a woman's hair is a glory to her. As children of God and representatives of Christ, we can present Him to our world in a more appealing way when we are well groomed. Each of the areas we cover in this book is important in helping us look our best. However, clean, styled hair certainly plays a larger part than pedicured toenails!

Hair, much like skin, is made up of three layers. (*See* Figure 7-1.) The cuticle is the outer layer. It has tiny scalelike cells that point downward and protect the inner layer. The cortex, or inner layer, is a fibrous substance with long cells. Its job is to give elasticity and strength to the hair. The cortex also contains the pigment that gives your hair color.

Hidden away in the center of the hair shaft is the medulla. The medulla gives the hair strength and thickness. The medulla is often missing in fine hair but is abundant in thick hair. It takes a stretch of your imagination to envision that each single hair has all three of these parts, but they are there. And they need to be cared for.

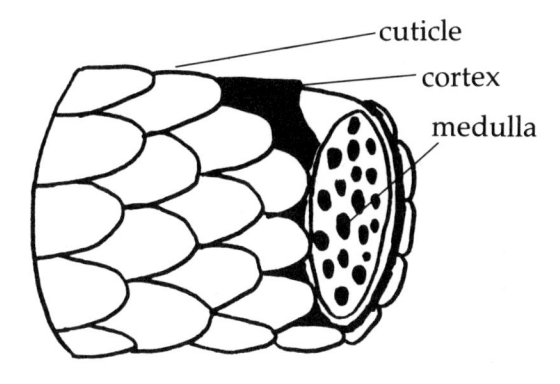

Figure 7-1. Hair Cross Section

Basic Care

Shampoo

Shampooing, the first step in effective hair care, is the key to clean, shiny hair. The shampoo you choose is important, and it's more effective if it matches your hair type: dry, normal, or oily; and your hair texture: fine, medium, or coarse. Look for the PH balance indicator of 4.5 to 6.5 on the label of your shampoo. Many shampoos now have sun-protection ingredients, such as PABA, to prevent sun damage to your hair. These should be listed on the label as well.

There are so many brands of shampoos. Bright, slick slogans and pretty packaging try to convince us that one is better than the other. These tactics sometimes work on me, too!

You can find several very good shampoos at a beauty-supply store. I prefer to use professional hair-care products as opposed to supermarket types that can be high in detergent and high in alkali. Beauty-supply-store brands may be a few dollars more, but they are worth it to me because I know that the products I am using are not damaging my hair.

If you do use a detergent shampoo, store half of it in another container, fill up the original bottle with water, and shake it vigorously. The half-shampoo, half-water mixture weakens the detergent. It also makes the shampoo last longer.

Special-feature shampoos, such as those with henna added, are for specific results. Henna shampoos used on medium-brown and brunette hair tones add shiny red-toned highlights to your hair. Anti-dandruff shampoos reduce flakiness and treat the dandruff condition. Speaking of dandruff, dry scalp is often confused with dandruff. They are not the same. If your hair (or scalp) is dry you can treat it with hot oil treatments, proper shampooing, diet, and scalp massage. Massaging your scalp stimulates blood circulation and oil-producing glands in the skin which nourish the dry scalp. Massaging is also relaxing! Dandruff, however, needs a medicated shampoo. See your dermatologist if you discover anything on your scalp that you suspect is not healthy.

Depending on the amount of oil in your hair, shampoo every day or every other day. Greasy hair looks darker, separates, and is unappealing. Greasy hair can easily be avoided with regular shampooing. Besides, clean hair responds better to curling and styling!

Put a quarter-sized drop of shampoo in your palm. Rub it between your hands and apply evenly throughout your wet hair. Use your fingertips, not nails, to work the shampoo all the way to the roots. Don't forget your hairline and the nape of your neck. Shampoo twice if your hair is especially oily or dirty.

Next, rinse your hair with warm water through and through until the last trace of shampoo disappears. Run your fingers through your hair while you are rinsing it so that the water from the shower nozzle can run through it. If you do this regularly your hair should be clean, shiny, and manageable. If it isn't, try changing shampoos.

When the shampoo is all rinsed out, you are ready for step number two: conditioners and rinses.

Rinses

Rinses are used right after shampoo. Normal hair rarely needs a special rinse. Dry, fine hair needs a professional cream rinse; oily hair needs an acid rinse to cut down on the oil. One-half cup of apple cider vinegar mixed with two cups of water is a good rinse for oily hair. It also cuts through shampoo, conditioner, setting lotion, mousses, and hair spray buildup. Use the vinegar rinse on normal and dry hair once a month. Be sure to rinse the vinegar mixture out of your hair. To make it more convenient, premix the solution and keep it in a plastic bottle near your shower.

I keep all of my hair-care products, a razor, soap, bubble bath, shower cap, shaving cream, body exfoliating cream, and massage mitt in a decorated basket. That way I can carry it to the bathroom when I shower or bathe. You may want to do the same.

For you blondes who have swimmer's hair—that green tint—try using a rinse made with one tablespoon of baking soda dissolved in one cup of warm water. Use after you shampoo. This will strip off any residue left on your hair. If your hair is already affected by chlorine and is tinted, a quick rinse with tomato juice will counteract the effects of the chlorine and get the green out.

Conditioners

Conditioners are available in both deep-penetrating and instant types. Deep-penetrating conditioners work their way into the hair strand to moisturize and nourish. An instant conditioner is applied on hair ends where you need it. Your roots rarely need conditioner. Using conditioner on your roots just causes your hair to get oily. Instant conditioners actually coat the hair strand with a waxy substance, making your hair manageable and tangle free, but they also often make your hair too soft and less curly. Use more or less instant conditioner to suit your own hair. Avoid products with beeswax in them.

A deep conditioner is supposed to be left on your hair for five to fifteen minutes before you rinse it out. Most deep conditioners work better if you wrap your head in a hot, damp towel or sit under a hooded hair dryer for about ten minutes. This causes the conditioner to penetrate deeper. Use deep conditioners once a month on normal hair, more often on colored, damaged, permed, or dry hair, maybe two to three times a month. Oily hair rarely needs a deep conditioner except perhaps after a chemical process such as a permanent.

A Cut Above

Hair grows about one-half inch per month, varying, of course, from person to person. There is little you can do to make your hair grow faster. You can try heavy brushing, which stimulates your blood circulation. This can encourage growth. Balanced eating, exercise, and sleep also help you grow healthy hair.

Trimming your hair doesn't make it grow, as you may have heard. It does, however, keep it healthy, full, and tidy looking. It also eliminates split ends.

Split ends occur when the first two layers of the hair strand—cuticle and cortex—wear away because of hair dryers, curling irons, hot rollers, and other kinds of abuse. This leaves the medulla's fine milklike strands to split. If the ends are not cut off, the split will continue up the hair strand, leaving it thin, frizzed, and weak. No product can solve the split-end problem, though many claim to. Split ends must be cut off regularly.

Your hair should be trimmed every six to eight weeks, which will put an end to split ends and help retain the shape of your hairstyle. Trim your hair every four weeks if you are trying to change your hairstyle or correct a problem.

Your haircut and style are high-ranking factors in hair care. A good cut can make all the difference. A good cut is dependent upon a good hairstylist.

Choosing a Stylist With Style

Your hairstylist needs to be a professional who cares enough to take time to get to know you and to learn your hair likes and dislikes. You will benefit most from a stylist who understands the art of custom hair design. You don't want a mass-produced haircut. Get a design that fits you. It may be a style similar to someone else's, but because each face is different, your hairstyle should be trimmed and tailored just for you.

Take a photo into the hair salon with you so your stylist will have a better idea of the look you want. You can even stop by the salon to discuss hairstyle before you make the appointment. Decide whether or not your hair texture can actually achieve the style you have in mind. Be realistic, and remember, it will never turn out exactly like the picture!

If you see someone with a haircut you like, ask her who her stylist is! Also, if your hair looks better when your stylist does your hair than when you do it, ask him or her to teach you how to style your hair. Don't be shy—it's *your* hair.

I usually consider the condition and style of a hairdresser's hair before I let him or her cut my hair. This may be just my own quirk, but I want my stylists to care about their own personal appearance as much as they care about mine.

The Right Style for You

You have to wear your hair all the time, so here are several things you should consider before you choose a hairstyle.

Can Your Hair Handle It?

Is your hair actually capable of achieving the style you want? You can't force your hair to do what it can't! You will be happier with the results if you try styles that will work with your hair.

Personality and Life-Style

What is your personality and lifestyle? Bubbly girls usually don't wear long, sophisticated curls or fancy twists. Likewise, shy, reserved girls rarely turn up with hair that is spiked, shaved, or has uneven sides. Life-style is important, too. Girls who are active or involved in sports need a cut that is short and easy to care for, or a no-fuss shoulder-length style that can be pulled back out of the way. Elaborate, puffy looks won't do for on-the-go girls! On the other hand, if you're an early riser and a good time organizer, take a shot at a more complicated style.

My life-style and personality demand a versatile, fairly easy hairstyle. I prefer longer hair so I keep it about shoulder length so that drying and styling time is reasonable. This also gives me several styling options. So whether I am going to church, teaching a class, or going out for pizza, I'll have a style that fits the occasion.

A Style That Suits Your Wardrobe

Adjust your hairstyle not only to the occasion but also to your outfit. Certain hairstyles do look better with certain outfits. Punk, spiked hair doesn't fit a puffy lace dress. Fluffy locks of curls look out of place with faded jeans and an old jean jacket. Get the picture? Also remember to get a haircut that does not limit your dressing.

Does Your Hairstyle Fit Your Body?

Your body size is another consideration when you are searching for that perfect haircut. Have your cut balanced and in proportion with your height and weight. My friend Cari has very thick, full hair that looks good with her height. If Cari were shorter and small boned, her hair would overpower her. Just the opposite is Kelli, who is shorter and heavier. Kelli wears her hair short but in a curly, full style. If she had a straight, flat style, it would make her body look bigger. The best style for her would be longer hair, but she prefers it short. That's okay as long as she keeps it full so that her head doesn't look small for her body size.

What Is Your Face Shape?

The next thing to consider is your face shape. I saved this one for last because it needs some explanation. There are millions of different face shapes but only seven major shapes, one of which we all come close to: oval, round, square, pear, heart, rectangle, and oblong or diamond.

Most people are a combination of two categories. To say that you have a square-pear face sounds pretty strange. I really don't care for these labels per se. I like to think I have a unique, one-of-a-kind face, which is exactly what I have. (So do you!)

The cosmetology (hair and makeup) world puts face shapes into categories. We have already discussed how makeup techniques have been designed to give every face an oval appearance. The same holds true for hair design. Most stylists will try to give you a cut that hides features which take away from that so-called perfect oval. Finding a style to complement your face shape is certainly valid, but trying to change your face shape with a hairstyle is insulting the creativity of God. He made us all so individual. Select a style you enjoy and feel good in—a style that lets you be you!

As I said, there are certain styles that will complement you more than others. There is a general guideline to keep in mind which applies to hair as well as to clothing necklines (which we will talk about later). The guideline is this: Try not to repeat your face shape with your hairstyle. Very easy. If you have a round face, stay away from a super curly and short style. Try a longer, straighter look. For a square face, keep your curls or fullness away from the corners of your forehead and jawline. An oblong face looks best in a style that is full at the cheekbone and no longer than the base of your neck. Are you getting the picture?

On the pear-shaped face, rather than repeating the fullness of the jaw and the narrowness of the forehead, do the opposite—curls or waves on top and smoothness near the jawline. If you have a heart-shaped face, save the fullness for your chin area. And those of you who are convinced that diamonds are forever, just avoid fullness in the cheekbone area.

Long Neck or Short Neck?

When deciding on how long to wear your hair, consider your neck length also. Short necks are complemented by shorter hair. Long necks look good either way, in my opinion. Most hairstylists would encourage girls with long necks to wear longer hair. I agree. But I have seen long, thin-necked people with very short hair, and it looks great. So the best rule is this: To each her own!

Types of Cuts and Terms

To help you feel more confident, and able to speak with knowledge to your stylist, here is a list of common haircuts with brief definitions.

Blunt. Hair is cut so that all the ends, when combed straight down, are even and level with each other, the way a paintbrush is cut. (See Figure 7-2.)

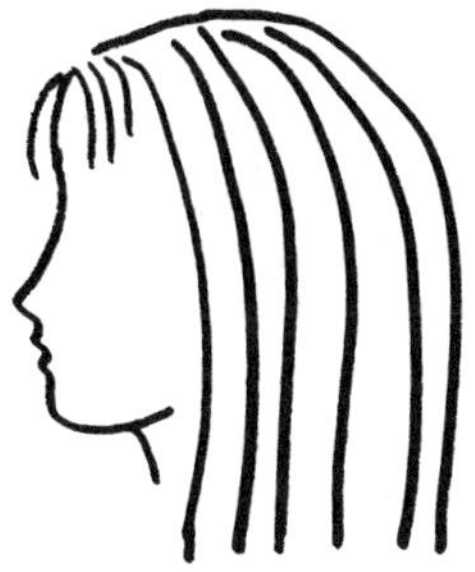

Figure 7-2. Blunt Cut

Beveled. This is slightly similar to a blunt cut, except that the hair either underneath or on top is a tiny bit shorter. This helps the hair bend under or look fuller on short styles, like a wedge cut. (See Figures 7-3a, 7-3b.)

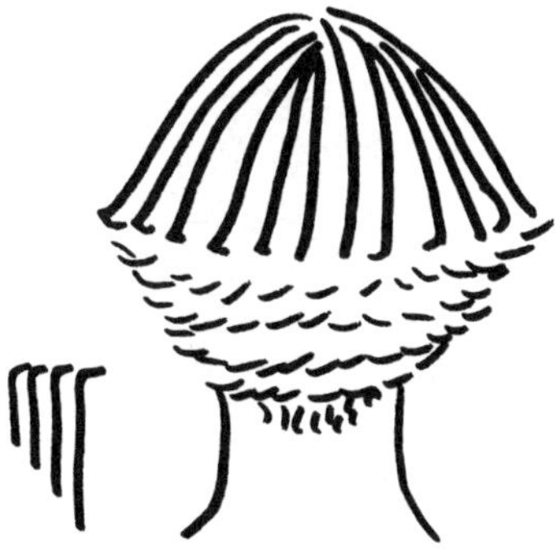

Figure 7-3a. Beveled Cut

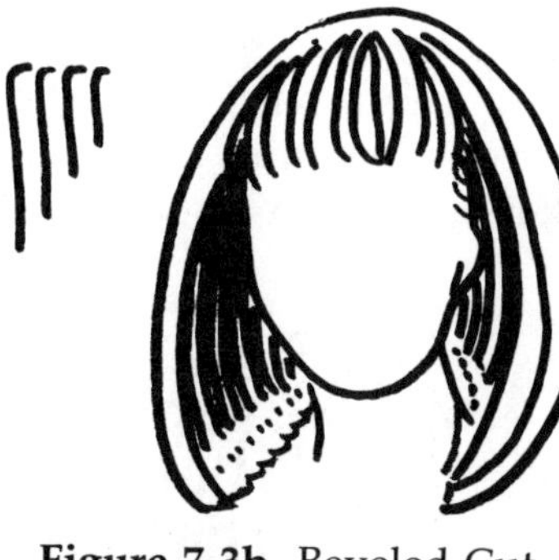

Figure 7-3b. Beveled Cut

Layered. Hair is cut so it will fluff and have more fullness. It is shorter on top and gradually achieves more length in the back. This creates fullness on top, yet retains length. (See Figure 7-4.)

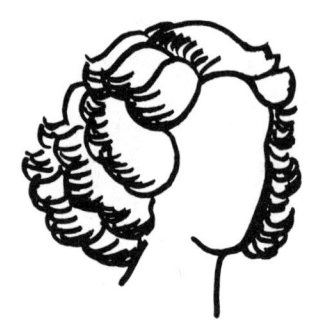

Figure 7-4. Layered

Tapered. This is a short haircut in which the hair at the nape of the neck is cut very short and gradually gets longer and fuller at the crown area. The same cut can be applied to the sides above the ears, too. (*See* Figure 7-5.)

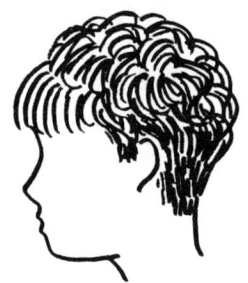

Figure 7-5. Tapered

Bi-level. This is a drastic change in the lengths of hair from sides to back to bangs. Usually this is used with a drastically short haircut at the sides and a long, sometimes blunt cut at the back. *Bi* means "two"—two levels. (*See* Figure 7-6.)

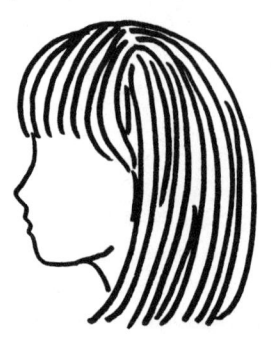

Figure 7-6. Bi-level

Undercut. This can refer to two different looks. First, the hair is cut so that it will scoop under naturally or more easily when it is curled. The second is when the hair is long but a small amount right at the nape of the neck is cut to add interest when the long hair is worn up off the neck. (*See* Figure 7-7.)

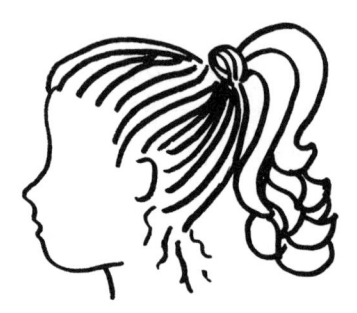

Figure 7-7. Undercut

Asymmetrical. The hair is not cut even on both sides. One side is cut shorter than the other side. This is generally done at a forty-five-degree angle, but can be more severe for a more dramatic look. (*See* Figure 7-8.)

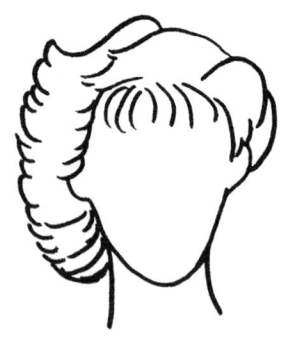

Figure 7-8. Asymmetrical Cut

Thinning. This means carefully cutting out sections of the hair to make it thinner. This is used primarily on extremely thick hair. Thinning has recently been used to "texture" the hair to give it a more lacy appearance. (*See* Figure 7-9.)

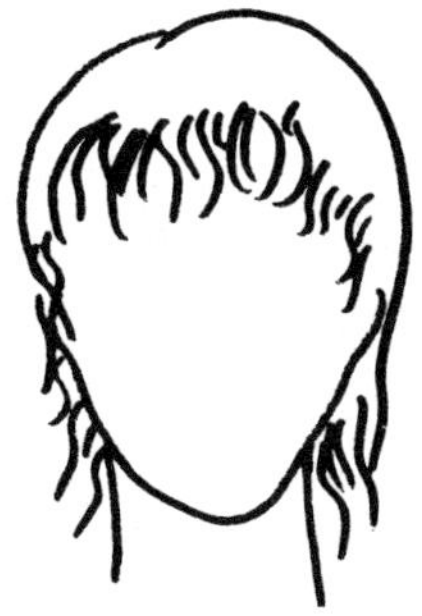

Figure 7-9. Thinning

Your sylist will adjust each type of cut to your needs. Remember to use your hairstyle to be yourself. You don't need to be a copycat! Hopefully your reason for wanting a certain style is not because you want to look like somebody else.

A young woman I recently met shared a personal insight with me. We were at a state fair, standing in line waiting to get hot cinnamon rolls—oh, yum! A guy was walking toward us who had his hair shaved in a Mohawk style. It was spiked down the center and shaved on the sides. He strolled up to me and asked if I had seen his friend. When he described his friend as a person with spiked bright-red hair I said no. I had not seen him. I was sure I would have noticed him if he had gone by. When the guy walked away, Sherri snickered. She told me that just a year ago she had been a punker and wore her hair spiked on one side. Sherri said she was trying to make a statement. But she realized she could be an individual without looking like that.

Hairstyles often become fads. Asymmetrical cuts, spiked hair, and whatever drastic style emerges on the scene are fad-type haircuts. These styles are more difficult to change if you have an extreme haircut. Be stylish instead of faddish.

An important note: Don't change your hairstyle based on your feelings or emotions on one particular day. Many times, if we have a bad day or are sad or just don't like ourselves too well, we decide that a drastic change in our appearance will lift our spirits and make us feel fresh and new. Well, maybe for a day or two! When the excitement wears off, we can be left with an unwanted look or hair color! Subtle changes in style are easier to handle. Take time when you make style-changing decisions.

I truly believe we females look our best when we have haircuts and styles that are feminine rather than boyish looking. God created us female and that is terrific! Even short boyish styles can have soft feminine touches.

Special Effects

The amount of wave—or lack of it—in your hair depends on its basic shape. You would need a microscope to see this, but it's true: your hair strands fall in one of three shapes: round, oval, or flat.

Round strands produce straight hair; oval strands result in wavy hair; flat strands will leave you with curly hair. You don't necessarily have all the same shape strands throughout your head. I have flat strands around my face—the curliness gives it away! The rest of my hair strands are probably oval shaped. When I was younger, my hair was extremely curly. I wasn't crazy about it then, but now I am glad I have a natural wave to my hair.

Our hair shape is given to us. I have found it is best to let my hair do its thing naturally rather than fighting it. I have learned to use my natural wave and medium texture to create soft,

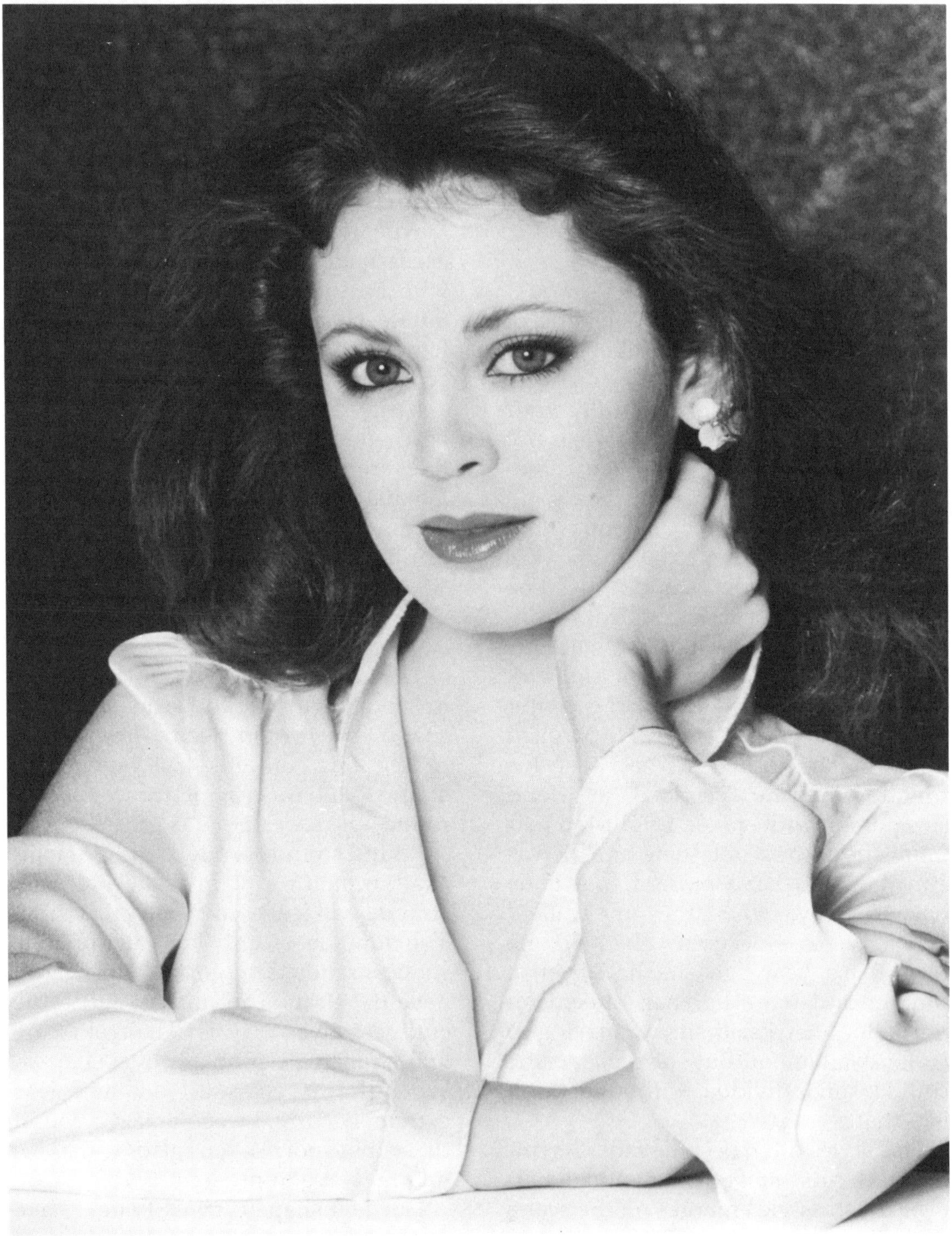

Figure 7-10. My hairline has a look all its own.   Photo by Keith Mead.

feminine styles. The straight-hair look was never meant for me.

What about you? Is your hair straight, wavy, or curly? Fine, medium, or coarse? Do you have any cowlicks or a widow's peak? My hairline is staggered and peaks a little right in the very center. I like the look it gives. (*See* Figure 7-10.)

Perms and Waves

Many girls want more curl in their hair, so they give it a little extra pizzazz with a permanent or body wave. Both of these procedures use a chemical solution that restructures your hair shaft into a new shape—an S shape. Perms may be very curly or mildly curly. It depends on the size permanent rod your stylist uses. Body waves use a larger rod to create a soft wave instead of a curl. Partial perms are usually done on the front or top hair only.

Relax!

Hair relaxers or straighteners do just the opposite of the perm or body wave. These products take the S shape out of your hair.

I recommend that you have these procedures done by a professional who has analyzed your hair and can select the type of perm, body wave, or straightener that will perform best on your hair.

The chemicals used can actually damage your hair, causing it to become dry, brittle, or frizzy. Usually it is better for your hair if you just work with what you have—your natural, untreated hair! Chemically treated hair needs to be cared for with kindness. Condition it regularly if it has been treated or colored. It needs the extra moisture.

A Splash of Color

Coloring, lightening, highlighting, weaving, and painting the hair are all ways of brightening up your look. Coloring your hair requires a dye that changes the hair pigment. Dyes are available in long-lasting or temporary forms. Temporary colors in spray cans or gels have become popular but will probably die down soon. They can be fun but are not normally worn for everyday occasions.

During the summer months my husband, Bill, a youth pastor, takes the kids on "beach day." I love going to the beach, so I always go with them when I can work it into my schedule.

One foggy valley morning, as we loaded the vans to head for the beach, along came Lindy with her blonde hair sticking straight up, a splash of red coloring spray right in the front—a bit off center. Though she was approaching us in her sophisticated, "Hey, I'm cool," strut, we couldn't help but chuckle to ourselves. The best part of the story happened at the beach.

Soon after we arrived, Lindy bravely charged into the ice-cold water. When she came out, streams of faded red color ran down her face. It was priceless. When the red faded away, so did Lindy's attitude. We spent the rest of the day enjoying Lindy just being herself!

Hair painting is a way to add temporary or semipermanent color the way you want it and where you want it. Many of these products can be purchased in your local drugstore. If you plan on temporarily coloring your hair by yourself, be sure the package says *temporary*. Semipermanent does not mean temporary!

If you are going to use these products, I have two suggestions: First, do a patch test before applying anything to your whole head! See how your hair will react and how the product will really look on you. Second, remember that these treatments must be well blended and must match your natural skin tones.

Just for fun, ask yourself why you want a perm, body wave, straightener, lightener, or a certain style. Do you want to look like so-and-so, or believe that blondes have more fun (it's not true)? Are you bored or upset, changing your hair color or style based on feelings? Think before you act. Discuss the decision with your hairstylist and your parents. The Lord made your hair color and skin tones to match perfectly. Unnatural coloring and chemical treatments can detract from your appearance.

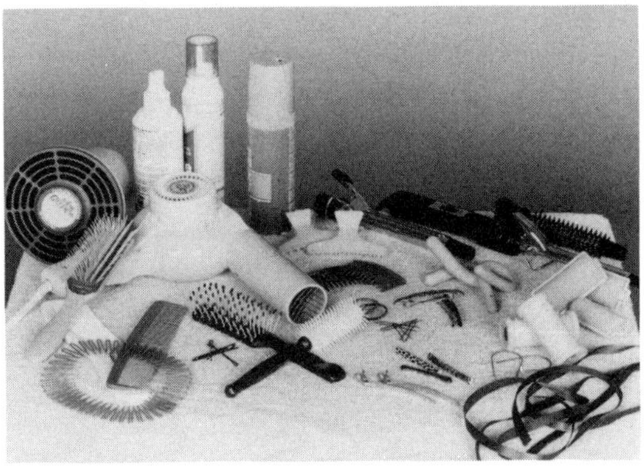

Tools and Techniques

There are several different tools that are a must in effective and controlled hairstyling. (*See* Figure 7-11.) There are also techniques that will help you to achieve the look you are after. Here is a brief description of some of them.

Combs

A handy tool indeed, and one of the most commonly used items in hair care. Combs are multipurposed—they smooth hair, part it, remove tangles, and style it.

Most combs have two sizes of teeth: wide and narrow. The wide-toothed end is for thick hair and for untangling hair, especially when it's wet. Always

Figure 7-11. These handy hair tools will keep your hair looking its best. Left to right: diffuser, dryer, hair spray, mousse, setting lotion, clamps, curling iron with larger and smaller rod attachments and curling brush, rubber-padded brush, combs, vented brush, round brush, decorative combs, twister curlers, sponge and hot curlers, bobby pins, hair pins, barrettes, duckbill clamps, ribbons.

begin at the ends of the hair, slowly working your way up toward the roots. It is a common mistake to start combing through wet hair at the root and pull the comb through the tangles. Ouch! This hurts your scalp and also your hair because you can't help but break and split it!

The narrow-toothed end of the comb is for refining and specific styling.

Rubberized combs are easier to work with because they flex with your hair. So, when you encounter a tangle, using a bendable comb can take care of it with much more ease.

Finger combing is a fun and carefree technique for hair that is short to short-medium in length. Simply towel dry your hair. Then begin working your fingers through your hair as you would work a brush or comb. Give it direction and lift. Repeat often until your hair is dry. Now lightly comb it and spray. You may not want to comb it at all!

Brushes

Brushes come in all sizes, shapes, and colors. Pocket-sized brushes are great for your purse, but larger brushes do a better job at styling. Round brushes are great for styling while you blow dry, but not practical for normal brushing. Round brushes don't work well on long hair. It is too easy to get long hair tangled in the brush.

The kind of bristles your brush has is important. Old-fashioned, less-expensive brushes, with the cluster nylon bristles, are harder on your hair and can cause tangles themselves. Your best bet is a brush with widely spaced, bendable bristles with rounded tips, set in a rubber pad. Test the bristles to see if they move easily. You want them to have some "give" so they won't break your hair strands.

Vented brushes are good for styling while you dry. They allow the warm air to flow through them directly to your hair.

Natural boar-bristle brushes are good for fine and medium-textured hair. This type of brush is known for its ability to distribute natural scalp oils throughout your hair.

Besides styling, distribution of oils is a main purpose of brushing. It keeps the scalp and hair shafts moisturized. A good scalp massage will do the same thing. Both scalp massage and brushing will stimulate oils from the scalp. Brushing, though, gets the oil from the scalp out to the ends of the hair.

Brushing adds shine, cuts down on flakiness, and encourages growth by increasing blood circulation in the scalp. Great nourishment. Beware—overbrushing can make your hair greasy or can cause it to break. The best time for thorough brushing is right before you shampoo. Then you get the benefits of brushing without the greasiness that may follow.

Keep your brushes and combs clean. Why use a dirty brush on shiny, clean hair? Wash brushes and combs in the sink or toss them into the washing machine, zipped in a laundry bag. It's easy. Do it regularly.

If static cling has taken up residence in your hair, here's a tip for making it move out! Gently rub your brush or comb with an antistatic sheet that your mom uses in the dryer so the socks don't stick to the shirts. Now, slowly brush through your hair. Good-bye, static cling. A light mist of hair spray brushed through your hair will often remove static cling, too!

Blow Drying

Blow drying has come a long way. Women used to sit for hours under hooded dryers or bonnet caps (they look like oversized shower caps) with a hose connecting them to the main drying unit. Hand-held dryers are much easier and much faster to use.

The time it takes to dry your hair depends on the speed and heat of the blow dryer. It also depends on your hair's texture and length. Fine hair and short hair dry faster. Coarse, thick hair and long hair take more time. Use the high speed only for drying very wet hair or for straightening hair. Keep the air moving continuously. Hold the dryer about six inches away from your scalp to prevent overheating or burning your hair.

The way you dry your hair can keep it from being damaged by the dryer's heat. Begin by drying the back, near your crown. Concentrate on the roots first, ends last. Blow your hair in the opposite direction from its natural growth to get more fullness in it. Reduce the speed and heat of the dryer when your hair is almost dry. Now is the time to use your round brush and/or fingers for styling. Twirl the ends around the brush to curl them. Let the hair on the brush cool for a minute before removing it from the brush. Work in the direction you want your hair to go.

Divide your hair into sections, styling one area at a time. Find out what works best for you. Some girls style the back of their hair first, others the front. My naturally curly hair goes crazy around my face, especially the bangs, if I don't style the front first.

Daily blow drying can be hard on your hair, making it dry and brittle. Using a protective spray on your hair can help cut down on possible heat damage. You can find a good protective spray or lotion at a beauty-supply store. Read the bottles to be sure you get the kind that is right for your hair: dry, normal, or oily. Spray it on before you begin drying.

Apply conditioning mousses and styling lotions before you begin drying. They, too, can help prevent heat damage. Many mousses contain alcohol, so check to see that the one you buy doesn't!

The best drying technique for your hair is air drying, the natural way. Give your hair a break and let it dry naturally as often as possible. A diffuser is a good compromise between natural drying and blow drying. A diffuser evenly distributes the heat and broadens the blast of air. This promotes any curl or wave you may have in your hair to do its thing!

Wash-and-go seems to be the easiest way to care for your hair; however, it usually doesn't leave you looking your best. This method can leave your hair looking lifeless and straggly. It depends on your hair, of course. You can give a better impression and look more attractive if you don't show up places with your hair wet. Get up earlier if you need to, or braid your wet hair to make it look styled. The exception to this is hair sculpting. This is a current technique in which you apply a sculpting lotion or gel to your wet hair. Then you style your hair and allow it to dry naturally. The gel holds the style in place. When it dries, it feels hard and crunchy, but if you brush it out, it feels soft yet still holds its style and shape.

Rollers

Curls, curls, and more curls. They add softness and give fullness and a new look to your hair.

There are two types of rollers most commonly used: electric or hot rollers and sponge rollers. Hot rollers are the easiest and quickest way to get the curl and fullness you want. You will get the best results when you use them on just-washed, just-dried hair. Use end papers or toilet tissue to cover the ends of your hair before you roll it. (See Figure 7-12.) This protects the ends from the intense heat and also guarantees an even, straight-ended curl. Bent, frazzled ends just won't do!

The amount of time you need to leave the rollers in depends on your hair length. Longer hair, because its weight can actually take out the curl, will need to be in the rollers longer. A good way to curl long hair and get fullness into it using hot rollers is to pull all the long hair up into a ponytail on top of your head. Secure it with a covered rubber band. Now put the hot

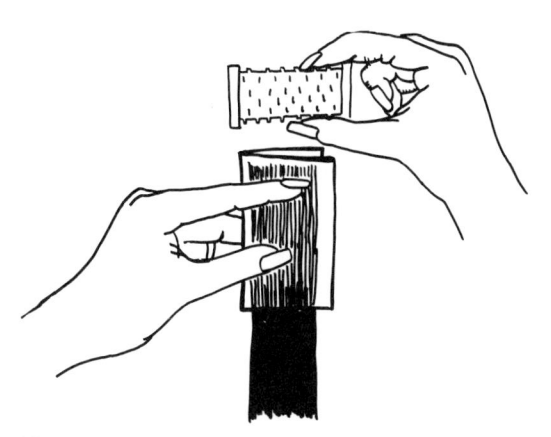

Figure 7-12. Cover ends of your hair with a tissue before rolling.

rollers any which way in the ponytail. When the rollers are cool, remove them and brush your hair for a full look. If you don't want a full look, only roll your curlers halfway up your hair. Do not use the ponytail method. Always give the rollers time to cool before removing them. The heat from the rollers weakens the hair, causing it to curl to the shape of the roller. If the roller and hair are not cooled off when you remove them, the curl may come out. If you are after only a slight curl, great! Take the rollers out sooner.

Just like blow drying, daily use of hot rollers really wears on your hair. Alternate your styles so you curl your hair one day and perhaps put it in a chignon the next.

Sponge rollers are very gentle on your hair and can be used as often as you like. Because they are soft you can sleep on sponge rollers. You'll have to see what works for you—rolling your hair at night and letting it dry and curl as you sleep, or blowing it dry and putting in rollers and leaving them in for a longer period of time. Unlike hot rollers, sponge rollers don't give instant curl.

Whether you use hot or cold rollers in your hair, brush out the curl very thoroughly, then follow with a hot hair dryer to relax the roller separations. If you have taken the time to curl your hair, don't ruin the look with separations and unbrushed curls.

As a general rule, roll your hair in the direction you want it to curl—up, under, straight back, forward, or angled. (*See* Figure 7-13.) To get more body in your hair, roll it all the way to the roots, especially on the top. (*See* Figure 7-14.) You will get more fullness and lift if you roll it this way.

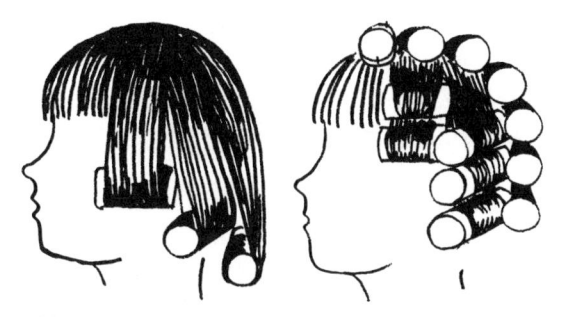

Figure 7-13. Roll hair in the direction you want the curls to go.

Figure 7-14. Rolling hair to the roots will give it more fullness.

Use different-sized rollers for different looks. Larger rollers give a bigger, looser curl. Small rollers create a tighter curl. For increased curl in a certain area, such as your bangs, use more rollers and a smaller size.

Bendable or twist rollers are the newest in hair curling. These brightly colored, flexible rods come in various sizes for various curls. Simply start at the ends of your hair, making sure they are flat against the roller. Roll all the way to the roots. Twist the ends of the rod toward each other so they stay in place. If they are preheated, leave them in for at least ten minutes. If cool, give them more time. Untwist them when you are done, fluff, and you have a head full of curls.

Curling Irons and Curling Brushes

For quick touch-ups, a curling iron comes in handy. Girls with short hair use this tool for touch-ups as well as overall curling. Some girls with long hair find it practical, some do not. Long hair gets more fullness from hot rollers.

Curling brushes are terrific for soft curls or adding a slight bend in the hair. This is what I use on my bangs when I wear the rest of my hair straight or pulled back. This type of brush is also great for calming shorter naturally curly hair, too. This makes for a more "organized" curl.

Many brushes and irons are sold together in kits with interchangeable parts, but they can be purchased as separates. Curling brushes and irons are definitely useful tools.

Clips and Clamps

Clips and clamps can be used to create curls or waves. Bobby pins are a small version of a clamp. They are used to secure a specific style such as buns, chignons, rolls, and twists. They are also used to create pin curls. Large pin curls leave hair wavy. Small pin curls leave hair with tight curls.

To make a pin curl, begin at the root of your hair. Wrap a small amount of hair around one to three fingers, depending on the tightness of curl you want. Then press the curl flat to your head. Put in the bobby pins, crisscrossed for a better hold. You can also use hair clips to secure the curl. Do this at bedtime for longer-lasting curls. If you are showering but not washing your hair, try curling it right before you get into the shower so the steam can moisten and encourage the hair to curl. Comb out after your hair is no longer moist.

Large duckbill clamps (the long, thin, silver ones) can be used on wet or damp hair to give a wavy look. Butterfly clamps do the same thing. Place the clamps in damp hair about one and one-half inches apart, all over your head. Let dry. Remove and brush. Follow with a light mist of hair spray. Experiment with the spacing of the clamps to get the wave you like best.

Simple Styles—Super Looks

The old commercial slogan about just washing your hair and not being able to do a thing with it doesn't have to be true for you.

There are countless numbers of styles for every hair type, texture, and length. Experimenting with styles lets you be creative.

Add decorative clips, barrettes, combs, ribbons, scarves, bandannas, even flowers and baby's breath to your hair to give it a special look. These accessories are not only attractive but they are also a great cure for the hairdo blahs. They are also cute ways of pulling your hair up away from your face so you can be seen. An upward sweeping given to your hair accents your cheekbone and eye area very nicely.

Many styling aids have popped up on the market in the last few years. Foamy mousse has become popular and effective for certain styles. Mousse, like setting gels or lotions, can be used before or after drying your hair. These products help give holding power and direction to your

HAIR HAPPENINGS

hair. Follow the instructions on the package carefully. Ask your stylist how you can use these products for your haircut.

Always choose high-quality hair aids. Many of them, including hair spray, are high in alcohol. If your hair had eyes, this would definitely make them water. Use a water-soluble hair spray. Use products your stylist recommends. High-quality products mean high-quality hair.

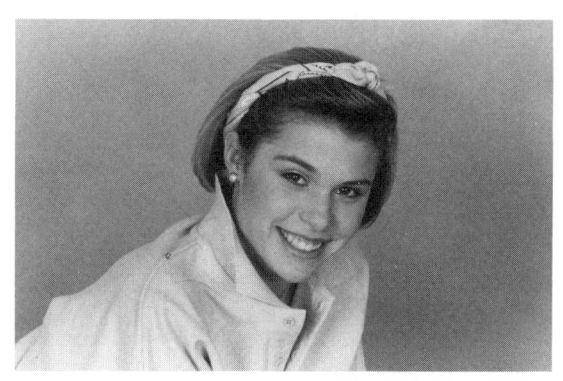

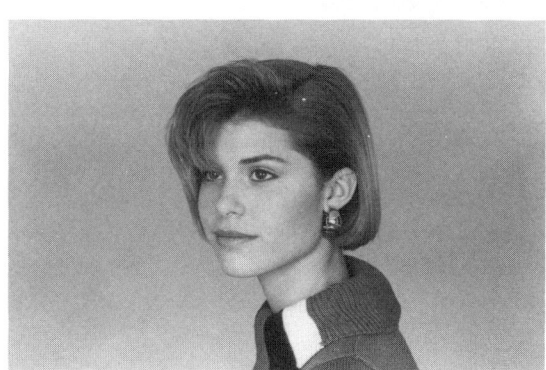

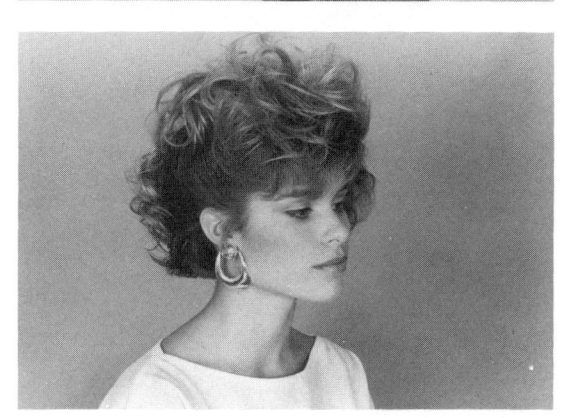

With a stretch of your imagination and a touch of creativity, you can come up with many cute and attractive styling ideas. Sporty, casual, high-fashion, holiday, sophisticated, wavy, curly, straight—the list goes on. Here are three quick and easy suggestions for the three basic hair lengths: short, medium, and long. These styles will work with most hair textures as well. Each of these styles changes your look just by changing your hair.

Figure 7-15.

Short and sporty. Comb your hair straight back, then tie a cute ribbon, bandanna, or headband around your head. Gently pull your bangs forward, creating a loose, puffed look. To add a wave, apply styling gel or mousse to your bangs. Pinch your bangs into the wave, using your fingers.

Figure 7-16.

Short and classic. Comb one or both sides of your hair smoothly behind your ears. Part your hair on the side or in the middle. To get a lift in your bangs, simply tease lightly. Add styling gel or hair spray to hold them in place.

Figure 7-17.

Short and dressy. Curl your hair all over your head, using a curling iron or hot rollers. When your hair is curled, run your fingers through it to separate the curls, creating more curls. Lightly tease to add desired lift. Now pull one or both sides of your hair up loosely. Secure, using a decorative hair comb, barrette, or bobby pins. Place curls over the bobby pins to hide them. Apply a mist of hair spray. This one is especially good for layered hair.

BEAUTIFULLY CREATED

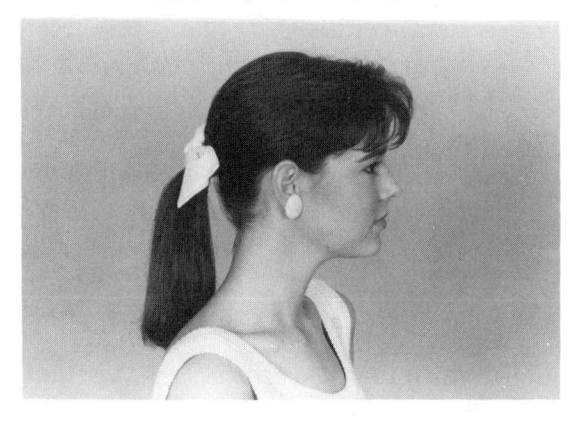

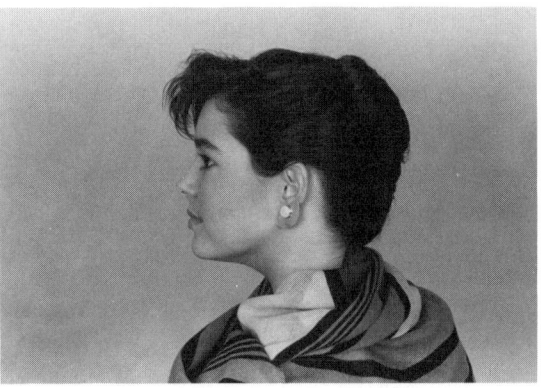

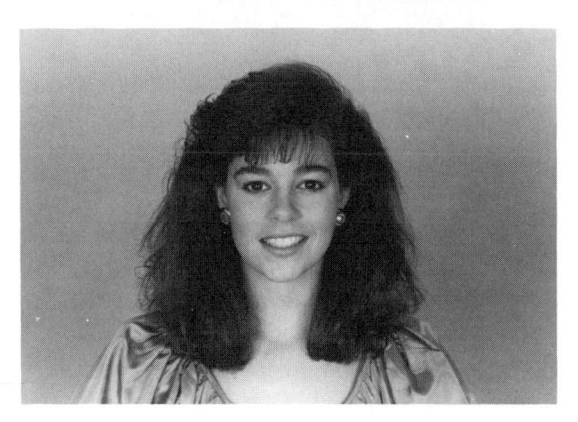

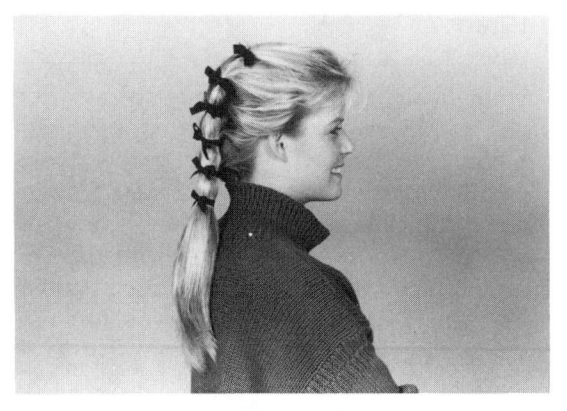

Figure 7-18.

Medium and sporty. Smoothly comb your hair back into a high or low ponytail. Fasten with a clip-on bow, barrette, or ribbon. Arrange your bangs. Tease lightly for a lift. Spray.

Figure 7-19.

Medium and classic. Comb all of your hair back and off to one side. Secure with bobby pins up the center of your head if needed. Now twist the rest of your hair in toward the center of your head, creating a roll. Tuck the ends of your hair in the twist or twist them into a chignon (bun). Secure with hair pins. (*See* Figure 7-24.)

Figure 7-20.

Medium and dressy. Roll your hair, using hot curlers. Roll the curler all the way to the roots, or pull hair up into a ponytail and roll the ends. When cool, remove the curlers and brush thoroughly. A little teasing just above your ears and near your bangs will add shape and fullness. Comb sides up and back, comb top of bangs at a slant, and add a few wisps of bangs on your forehead.

Figure 7-21.

Long and sporty. Pull your top section of hair into a ponytail. Secure, using a coated rubber band. Add another section to the first ponytail, an inch or so below it. Secure. Continue this process until all your hair is pulled back. Cover rubber bands with ribbons. Continue ribbons down the entire ponytail if desired.

HAIR HAPPENINGS

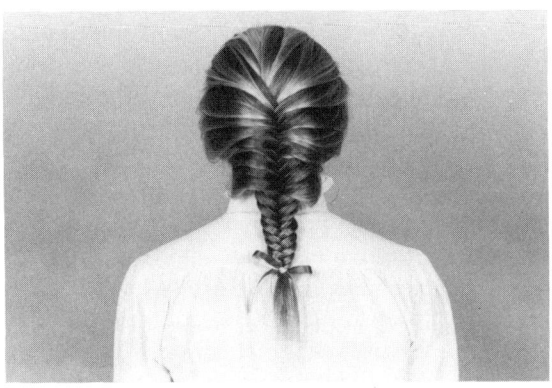

Figure 7-22.

Long and classic. This is called a fishtail braid. It is done with only two strands. Comb your hair straight back, then pick up two sections of hair at the top of your head. Cross them right over left. Now add a small amount of hair from the left side, above your ear, and add it to the section of hair you are holding on the right side. Repeat on the opposite side. Cross the two sections of hair again. Repeat these two steps until you reach the nape of your neck. You may stop here and make a ponytail, chignon, or add a bow. Or, to continue the braid, take a small amount of hair from underneath one section, bring it around and over, and add it to the opposite section. When you reach the end of your hair, secure and tug on the braid to even out the tension. Add a ribbon.

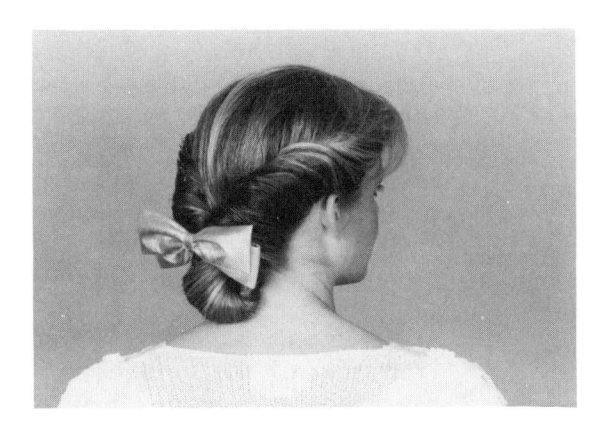

Figure 7-23.

Long and dressy. Brush one side of your hair up gently, then twist and tuck it into a roll. Hold it there with a barrette while you roll the other side. Pull the remaining hair together and twist it into a tight chignon. Bobby pin into place. Use hair pins or bobby pins to secure the two rolls. Cover the rubber bands and pin with a pretty bow.

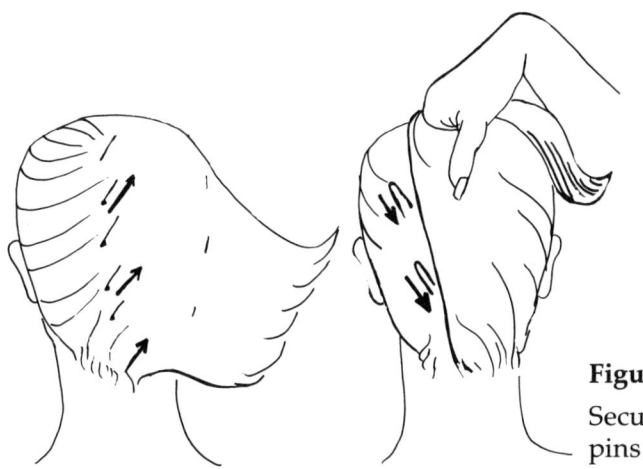

Figure 7-24.

Secure hair up the center, using bobby pins. Twist and pin. (*See* Figure 7-19.)

Tricks and Tips

1. First, I'll tell you my own pet peeve: uncovered rubber bands! Always cover over any rubber band or coated elastic band you wrap around a ponytail. You have so many cute and easy options available to you that look better than a bare rubber band. Take advantage of them. Keep a bag or box of colored ribbons, yarn, and thin scarves. Choose one that coordinates with your outfit and tie it around the elastic band. Barrettes or metal clips that have ready-tied bows on them are great, too. You might even want to try wrapping a section of your own hair around the rubber band. Take a section of hair out from underneath your ponytail. Wrap it around the rubber band. Secure the hair with a bobby pin under your ponytail. Now it looks more finished.

2. Back combing, also known as teasing or ratting, gives lift, volume, and control to your hair. And it gives it right where you want it. This should be done gently and sparingly. Overdoing back combing makes it look as if you have a bird's nest in your hair.

    Back coming is simple. Lift the section of your hair you are going to back comb. Hold it straight up, loosely. Now, starting near the ends, bring the comb down toward your scalp two to five times, or until you have achieved the lift you want. Smooth the hair over the teased area. I use this method occasionally at my crown and on the sides above my ears to lift my hair away from my face. *Please note:* Overly fluffy hair does not look right on young girls for everyday wear. Save it for a dressy occasion.

3. The next tip will save you from the frustration of barrettes and hair accessories that want to slide out of your hair. Fasten them in the opposite direction that your hair is going. This usually gives the barrettes, bobby pins, and decorative hair combs a tighter grip.

    To help hold decorative combs in place, bobby pin the ends of the comb. Do this underneath your hair so it can't be seen.

4. This trick adds a sleek look to your appearance: Create a neat loop with your hair by putting an elastic band around it as if you are making a ponytail. On the last wrap around with the band, only bring your hair three-quarters of the way through, leaving the ends of your hair wrapped in the elastic band. Now tie a ribbon around it. This is a great alternative if your hair is layered and won't fit into a smooth-looking bun or chignon.

5. This next tip is one you may have already discovered. It is the perfect solution to hard-to-handle hair. Lightly misting your style with hair spray will help avoid a stiff look, yet, once in a while a piece of flyaway or stubborn hair refuses to stay where you put it. Just spray a cotton ball with hair spray and dab in directly on the stubborn spot.

6. I occasionally see barrettes and combs just stuck in girls' hair for no reason. This looks awkward. Use these decorative tools to hold some part of your hair.

7. Holiday is a great dress-up time. For a good holiday look, use gold or silver ribbons or headbands. Rhinestone hair accessories are a nice touch, too. Wearing them for that special occasion will give you the right look.

8. Use a cute hat or sun visor as a hair accessory, and protect your skin at the same time! Sunglasses can be used in place of a headband for daytime.

9. Your bangs should be cut at an

angle, never straight across. Angled bangs look more natural and give a softer styling look. The center of your bangs is above your eyebrows. The shortest point, angle down evenly on each side.

10. Experiment with your part. Don't feel limited to wearing your part in the same place. Side, middle (when your bangs are in the front), slightly off center, even diagonal parts are stylish. How about no part! Discover a new look.

What Affects Hair?

Often when your hair is not responding the way it usually does, there is a reason. Incorrect shampoo or too much conditioner are two possibilities. Poor eating habits is another. Remember, you are not just satisfying your taste buds when you eat, you are feeding your entire body. Your hair is nourished through the blood circulating in your scalp. An unbalanced diet leaves your hair dull and lifeless. Inward care of your hair is as important as outward care.

Hormonal changes resulting from your menstrual cycle affect your skin, but did you know they can make your hair temperamental, too? The effect varies, depending on your hair and body chemistry. Dryness, oiliness, less curl, tighter curl, or total limpness are all possible reactions.

Stress, the topic of the eighties, can also be reflected in the condition of your hair. Drastically changing hair response or loss of hair can be stress related.

You can see that your hair, even though it has no feeling, can be directly affected by what goes on in your body.

The One Who Cares About Your Hair

"Are not five sparrows sold for two cents? And yet not one of them is forgotten before God. Indeed the very hairs of your head are all numbered. Do not fear; you are of more value than many sparrows."

Luke 12:6, 7

What do you think the point of these verses are? Do they mean that God is into hair counting? Maybe He can't believe all the hair we leave lying around. Maybe there's only so much hair to go around, so He has to ration it out.

Seriously, these verses are given to us to emphasize the fact that God never forgets about us. Each day we lose fifty to eighty hairs. That sounds like a lot, but nevertheless, the Lord knows exactly how many hairs we have at every moment. He knows even the most minor details about us—the number of hairs on our heads. If you lost forty-seven hairs today, would you know it? I'm not sure I would. Yet God does. His concern over our lives proves we are very valuable to Him. We matter to God in a very special way. His eyes and heart are turned continuously toward us. What can our response to this kind of love be?

An honest effort to be our best and look our best for Him is a good start. As children of God we represent Him. Our actions and our appearance speak louder than words. We have the privilege to style our hair and groom our appearance in such a way that it honors our heavenly Father. After all, He is the One who cares about every detail of our lives—even our hair.

HAIR HAPPENINGS

Project Page

1. Get to know your hair. Is it:
   - _____ dry
   - _____ oily
   - _____ normal
   - _____ combination
   - _____ dandruff
   - _____ fine
   - _____ coarse
   - _____ medium
   - _____ straight
   - _____ curly
   - _____ wavy

2. Now that you've identified your hair type, which type of the following products is best for your hair?
   shampoo_____
   conditioner_____
   rinse_____

3. What is a split end? How can split ends be minimized?
   _____
   _____
   _____
   _____

4. To determine the best hairstyle for you, describe each of the following about yourself:
   a. what your hair wants to do naturally_____

   b. your personality_____

   c. your life-style_____

   d. your style of dress_____

   e. your body shape and size_____

   f. your forehead——high or low?_____

   g. your face shape_____

   h. your neck length_____

   Now describe the hairstyle that fits you._____
   _____
   _____

HAIR HAPPENINGS

5. Using the various tools and techniques, tricks and tips given in this chapter, try four new hairstyles. Have a friend take a photograph of each one. Compare the photos to see which styles you look best in. Be creative!

6. Create your own hairstyle for each occasion: school, church, prom, movies.

7. Complete this sentence: Five things that affect hair are_____
   _____
   _____
   _____
   _____

8. God is concerned with the details of your life. List some of those details here._____
   _____
   _____
   _____

9. As children of God we represent Him. What are some hairstyles and outfits that do not honor God?_____
   _____
   _____
   _____

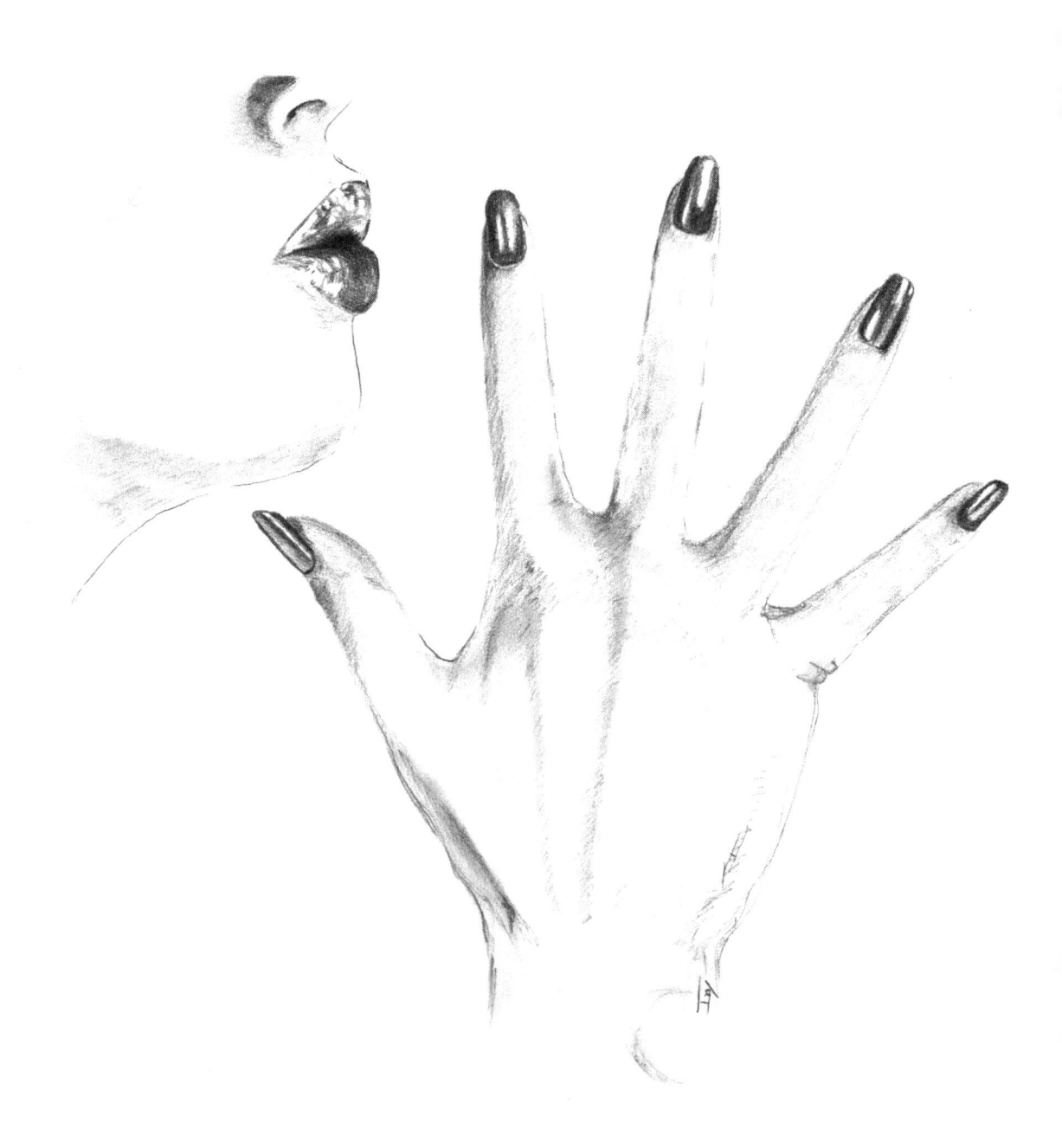

Figure 8-1.

8 HANDS AND NAILS
Nurtured to Perfection

Hands are constantly on the move. Writing, scratching, pulling weeds, playing sports, painting, baking, washing—the list goes on. And of course, everywhere our hands go, so do our nails!

Nails let us know when we have been ignoring them. They break, split, and chip. We get hangnails from dried-out cuticles and surrounding skin. Well-cared-for nails can make our hands and fingers look longer and more graceful. Short, stubby nails may be a sign of a nail biter or a nail picker, unless, of course, you keep your nails short for some practical reason such as sports, piano playing, or typing. I play the guitar, so the nails on my left hand are usually a little shorter than the ones on my right hand.

A weekly manicure helps keep your nails looking healthy and lovely. Even stubborn, hard-to-grow nails, or weak, thin nails, benefit from a manicure. If you feel embarrassed about your nails, a good manicure will help lift your spirits. You don't have to spend a whole evening on your nails, but do allow a minimum of thirty minutes for the whole process. Put on your favorite music tape and make your manicure an experience you enjoy.

What You Will Need

Collect the items you'll need before you begin. Lay them out on a hand towel to protect the tabletop from polish and polish remover.

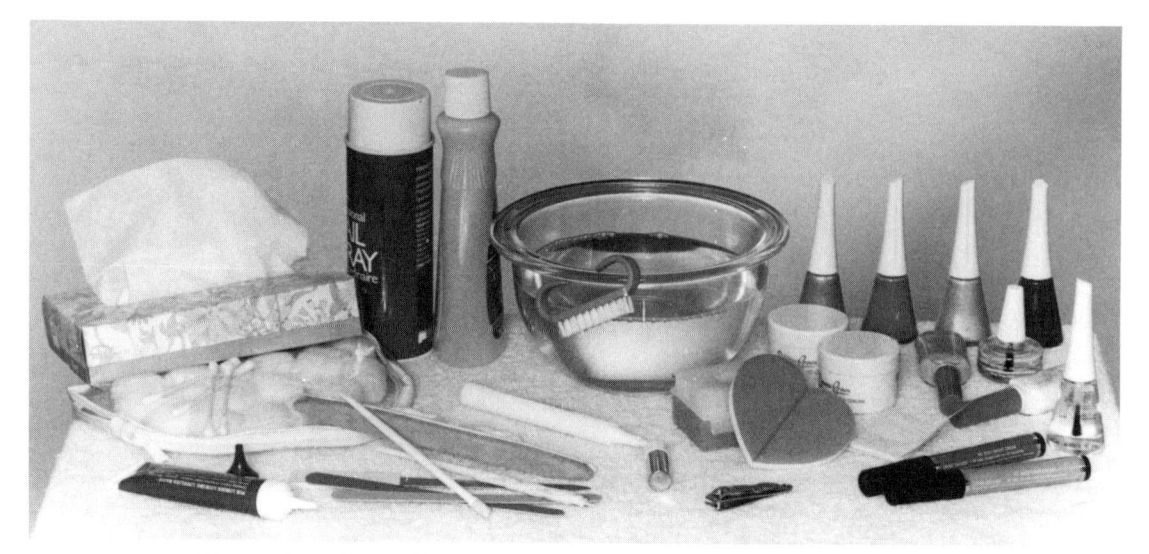

Figure 8-2. Everything you need for a magnificent manicure.

If you plan to do a professional job, round up cotton balls, cotton-tips, a dish of warm, soapy water, nailbrush, oily polish remover, emery board, nail clippers, orange stick, cuticle remover cream, nail buffer, buffing cream, base coat, clear nail hardener, polish, top coat, nail oil, and hand lotion. If you have a ripped nail, have a repair kit handy, too. (See Figure 8-2.)

Sounds as if you need a suitcase to gather it all up, but you won't! I store all of my nail products in a large clear zipper-top cosmetic bag. That way they're all together when I need them.

Manicure Magic

Going through a complete, detailed manicure step-by-step is the best method for learning how to care for your nails. Though this may seem complicated, once you catch on it will be a cinch!

1. Wet a cotton ball or tissue with oily nail polish remover. Press it gently on your nails for five seconds, then wipe off all old polish. Try using a remover-dipped cotton-tip to reach remaining polish along the edges of the nail.
2. Shape your nails in an oval. Square nails make your fingers look boxy, and pointed ones are bound to break! Use the rough side of an emery board and file from the side of your nail toward the center. Let the outer corner grow straight up a fraction of an inch, then angle toward the center. (See Figure 8-3.) This makes your nails stronger and less prone to ripping. Never saw back and forth! File in one direction or you'll force the nail dust down between the nail layers and they will split.

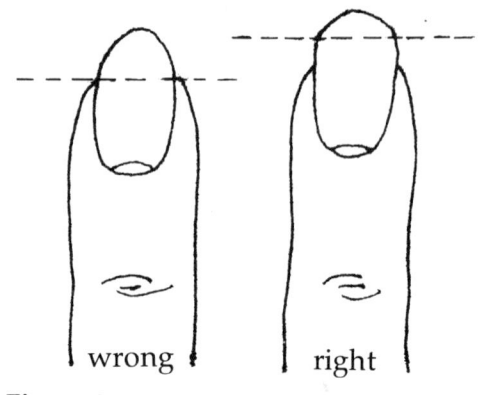

Figure 8-3.

Never cut your nails with scissors. Use clippers if you need to shorten, even out, or preshape your nail. When your nails are a nice oval shape, finish off the edges with the fine side of the emery board.

The length of your nails depends on (1) your activities, (2) how fast your nails grow, and (3) personal preference. Keeping your nails short may be practical, although they do make some fingers look stubby. Long nails are more prone to breaking and can look like claws if they get out of hand!

Medium-length nails are attractive, stronger, and easier to work with. Rarely do my nails grow longer than one-eighth inch over the *ends* of my fingers. Until my thirteenth birthday, I picked and bit my nails. Then my dad gave me a star sapphire ring with a small diamond on each side. When I slid the ring on my finger I thought, *This pretty ring just can't be on a hand with bitten nails.*

If it's hard for you to stop biting your nails, try brushing on one of those awful-tasting nail biters' products. It will help keep your fingers out of your mouth. Also, ask the Lord to help you have self-control. You will like the results.

3. Soak the ends of your fingers in warm, soapy water for two minutes to loosen and soften the cuticle and surrounding skin. Take a few deep breaths for relaxation while you wait.
4. Apply cuticle remover cream to your cuticle and gently massage it in. It doesn't actually remove the cuticle; it prepares the cuticle to be pushed back so that it is less noticeable. Use an orange stick wrapped with cotton to gently push the cuticle back toward the knuckle. Never cut your cuticle off. The cuticle is there to protect the nail base from infection. Always keep your cuticle well moisturized with hand lotion or night cream for nails. If dry, cracking cuticles are an ongoing problem for you, try soaking your nails nightly in warm olive oil. Pat the excess off—don't wash it off!
5. Scrub your nails with a soft-bristle nailbrush or toothbrush dipped in warm, soapy water. Rinse and pat dry.
6. Clip away any hangnails. Be sure you don't clip too closely and create a sore. Your skin is delicate.
7. Buff your nails. This helps them grow and gives them added strength and a smoother surface. The buffing action stimulates blood circulation, which nourishes and encourages growth. It also allows the protein or collagen in the buffing cream to penetrate the nail. Rough ridges are gradually smoothed out as well.

Apply a good buffing cream to your entire nail. Using a deerskin or other high-quality buffer, buff across your nail in one direction (away from you), using the full length of the buffer. Continue until buffing cream is gone and a natural shine develops. Rescrub your nail to remove buffing residue. Keep your buffer clean by wiping it with a clean towel after each use. I know buffing takes time, but it is the best treatment for weak, thin, slow-growing nails.

8. Seal your nails by brushing on base coat. Be sure your nails are dry. Many girls like to stop at the base coat. The shiny, clear look is very appropriate for daytime wear or for busy schedules. Base coat applied before polish will keep your nails from turning yellow from the polish.

If your nails are weak, you can use clear nail hardener or strengthener instead of base coat and nail color. There are strengtheners with fiber threads in them that are effective. A good nail strengthener that you don't rub on is gelatin, but you need to take it daily for several months before you will see any results. Gelatin comes in capsules or powder that can be added to fruit juice.

When I was preparing for the Miss Oklahoma Pageant, I needed to keep my nails hard and strong because, if one broke, it would throw off the sound of the guitar piece I was planning to perform. So, I would add one package of unflavored gelatin to one can of heated diet soda (orange, cherry, or strawberry) and put it in the refrigerator to harden. It made a pretty good low-calorie gelatin that enhanced my figure as well as my nails!

9. To paint or not to paint, that is the question. If you choose to go for it, apply one or two thin coats of polish. Allow the first coat fifteen to thirty minutes to dry completely before you add the second. This prevents smudges and dent marks. Use the three-stroke method—once down each side of the nail, then once down the middle. Be sure you coat the edge of your nail tip, too!

Keep harmony in your overall coloring by selecting nail colors in the same family as your blush and lip gloss. This creates unity and a more together look. (*See* Figure 8-4 in the color section.) Light colors are more appealing and graceful looking. They also make chips less noticeable. Dark polishes make the nails look heavy and smaller. Brush applicators provided with bottled polishes are good. Make sure to keep the cap tightly closed between applications. When polish becomes thick, add thinner or buy a new one.

Polishing pens often get sticky and out of control, but they are easy to use.

If you are going to wear nail polish, be responsible with it. As soon as it begins to chip off, reapply more polish or take it all off. Do not peel the polish off your nails! You can damage your nail by accidentally pulling off its top layer. Carry either remover or polish in your purse to avoid the temptation to pull off your polish.

Decorative polishing such as stripes, polka dots, or design stick-ons are fun, but they are also trendy and should be used sparingly. The same goes for glitter polishes and bizarre colors. Pretty, not putrid, is your goal.

10. Remove any polish you get on your skin or cuticle with a cotton-tip dipped in oily polish remover. A handy remover-filled pen with a sponge-tip applicator works well, too.

11. Now you are ready to apply a clear top coat or a clear nail hardener over the entire nail. Don't forget to brush some under the nail tip for added protection against chipping. Reapply the top coat the day after your manicure for a longer-lasting effect.

12. For the professional-looking finish with a well-moisturized touch, apply a small amount of thin nail oil on the cuticle area. Massage it in carefully. Take a look. Was it worth the time? Repeat your manicure weekly, adding or changing polish when necessary. Perhaps the best time to manicure is when you can allow a total drying time of thirty to forty-five minutes. This can be after homework is done, while watching TV, or right before bed.

Patching a Nail—the Painless Way

When your nail rips or tears near the edge, it is possible to save it. But if the rip is deep or long you might as well face it—the nail will have to go! When you trim the broken nail, be sure to trim all of your nails a little. To leave a few long and a few short looks unkempt and jagged.

Purchase a nail-repair kit that includes everything you will need. Follow the enclosed directions carefully. Be sure the fiber paper you adhere to your nails is flat—no wrinkles, creases, or air bubbles! Tear the paper off the sheet rather than cutting it. This will blend in more naturally with the nail surface. Always apply polish over repaired nails. Nail glue is handy, too. Just don't get it on your skin—you'll be stuck together for hours!

These nail-repair methods never really heal the rip, but they prolong cutting it off until the nail has grown longer. These methods will take some experimenting and practice to find the method that you like best.

Instant Nails

Whether you glue them on, press them on, or have them sculptured on, false nails should be only temporary. Your natural nails need to breathe to remain strong and healthy.

Fake nails on teens can look like dress-up. If you give them a try—whether it's to cover a torn nail that is growing out, even up a nail that is too short, or help you to stop biting your nails—use them on special occasions rather than for daily wear.

Glue-on and press-on nails have a tendency to pop off at the most inconvenient times. Sculptured nails get very expensive and require time-consuming trips to a manicurist.

Always follow directions for do-it-yourself nails and be sure to file them to a reasonable length. Forget about changing color unless you use polish remover without acetone. Of course, you can buy several shades of the prepolished type nail.

Beauty Tips for Nails

1. Wear rubber gloves when you need to have your hands in water for a prolonged period of time. Nails soften in warm water—not to mention the wrinkling effect on your fingertips.
2. Nails become brittle in cold weather, so wear gloves or mittens to keep them warm. (The fingerless gloves won't do it!)
3. Don't worry about the white spots under your nails. They are usually air pockets that form as your nail grows. Never fear—they eventually grow right out the top of your nail!
4. Keep an emergency nail kit in your locker, desk drawer, or purse.
5. Don't use your nails as tools to open envelopes and boxes, untie knots, remove staples, or pick trapped food from your teeth.
6. Protect your nails—especially if you have just polished them—by using a pencil to dial the phone. Pick up things with the pads of your fingers.

Helping Hands

Hands are our instruments of love. We greet each other, hug each other, and help each other with our hands.

In the Bible, we are referred to as God's hands and feet. This means we are used by God to reach out to others, expressing the Lord's love through our actions and touch.

Proverbs 31:20 teaches us that the Christian woman—young or old—is to extend her hands to the poor, and stretch out her hands to the needy. This woman cares what happens in the lives of others.

Jesus' hands healed, loved, comforted, and—most of all—were scarred for us. Jesus' nail-scarred hands provide forgiveness of sins, health, and eternal life for us today—right now. Open yourself up to being His instrument of love. Let your hands be like His.

Beauty Tips for Hands

1. Keep hand cream near your kitchen and bathroom sinks to use after you wash your hands.
2. Carry a tube of hand cream in your purse for on-the-spot use.
3. Wear rubber gloves when it's your turn to wash the dishes, mop the floor, or hand wash your delicate clothes or sweaters.
4. Use a rich, heavy cream or petroleum jelly on your hands at night, and wear white cotton gloves while you sleep.
5. Cotton gloves are also good protectors while you do housework or outdoor work. If anyone teases you about wearing gloves, tell him or her you're just giving the house the White Glove Test!

Fancy Feet

Even your feet, toes, and toenails need an occasional beauty treatment to keep them fun, fresh, and fancy looking. *Pedicure* is the technical name for a nail treatment on your toenails.

Follow the same steps on your toenails we outlined for fingernails, making adjustments where needed. Soak your feet in a basin or bathtub. Instead of filing toenails to an oval shape, simply cut them straight across. Then file to smooth out any rough edges. No need to ruin a pair of perfectly good nylons from rough toenails.

Apply polish only when your toes will actually be seen. Warm winter socks are not very revealing!

Feet have a tendency to get dry, chapped, calloused, and rough. Soak or cream your feet regularly to avoid these conditions. A pumice, loofah pad, or sloughing cream are all wonder-workers for removing dry, dead skin.

A little special attention, and your feet will feel refreshed and they'll step a little lighter!

HANDS AND NAILS

Project Page

1. What warning signals tell you that nails are being ignored? Which of these do you have? _____
   _____
   _____
   _____

2. Manicuring your nails once a week will keep them looking their best. For between-manicure nail treatments, keep a bottle of hand lotion next to the sink so you will have it handy to moisturize your cuticles and hands often.

3. Just for fun, get together with a friend. Take turns being the manicurist, giving each other a full manicure—and maybe even a pedicure!

4. Read Proverbs 31:20. List five ways you can lend your helping hands to your family, friends, church, and community in your daily activities. _____
   _____
   _____

5. Look up these Scriptures and match them to the way Jesus used His hands.
   a. Matthew 14:19 _____ to heal
   b. John 20:25 _____ to pray
   c. Matthew 9:29 _____ to die for us
   d. Matthew 19:13 _____ to feed the hungry

6. Read the following Scriptures and write down the way God tells us to use our hands.
   1 Timothy 2:8 _____

   Mark 16:18 _____

   Proverbs 31:13 _____

   Proverbs 31:20 _____

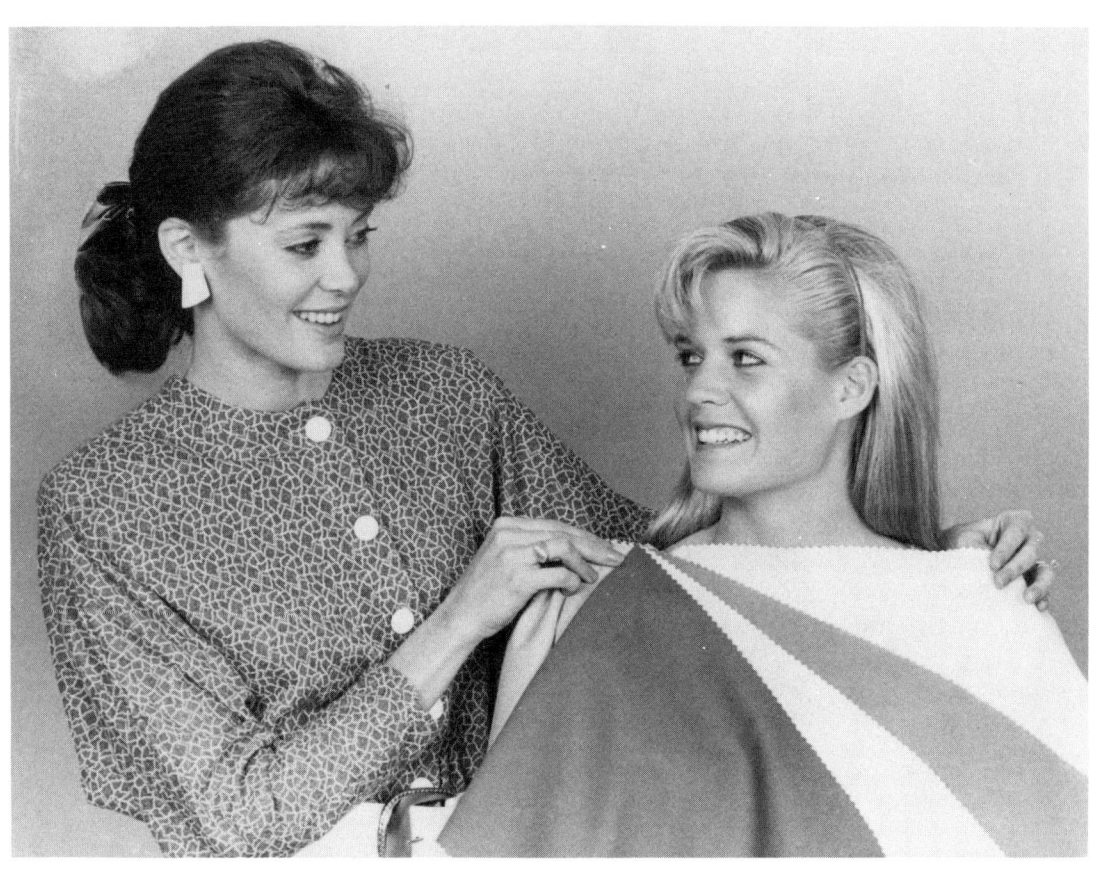

Figure 9-1. Using colored drapes is a good way to determine your color season.

9 DAZZLE YOURSELF WITH COLOR
Discovering Your Season and Colors

What colors do you look your best in? Which shades make your natural beauty dazzle? Does your skin seem to glow in some colors but appear drained in others? Discovering what colors work best with your natural coloring will give you a great new sense of presence and confidence.

Color analysis has become very popular. Perhaps you have had your colors "done," as they say. The idea of certain colors looking better on you than others is a valid theory. Your best colors will brighten your skin and accent your eyes. Correct colors will direct attention to you rather than to the color itself.

Nature divides color into four major seasons, and so do most accurate color theories. Smart idea! Who is the originator of color? Who thought up the brilliant idea of showering our world with beautiful hues? God did! Color was God's idea. And He lavishly splashed it in all four seasons—winter, summer, spring, and autumn—and in the rainbow.

There are no two people exactly alike, so it seems futile to try to lump everyone into four color categories: Summer, Winter, Spring, and Autumn. Yet, I would probably divide people into just two categories: cool and warm. Many people feel they have to stay in one color season, which is very restricting. Being divided into cool or warm allows you to choose colors from a broader range. For example, if you are cool you can choose colors from the Summer and

Winter seasons. Some colors may make you look better than others, but as long as they are cool, your appearance will be enhanced. Work within your undertone range and you will be doing well. Undertone? I'd better back up so you can get a complete look at this color craze!

Understanding the Seasons

When determining your color season, work with your natural coloring. Be open-minded! You may find out you look terrific in colors you've never worn before. Your "season" has nothing to do with the season you were born in or the time of year you like the most. Your season color category is determined by your skin, eye, and hair coloring, though the bottom line always comes back to your skin tone.

The tone of your skin comes from three pigments that are present in all skins, but in differing amounts: melanin (brown), carotene (yellow), and hemoglobin (red/blue). The special combination of these pigments in your skin gives you a unique coloring. Your skin tone is inherited and will not change. It will, however, deepen with a tan and fade with age. But since the undertone doesn't change, the same set of colors will always look good on you. (*See* the color section for sample color charts and seasons.)

Those of you with a blue-pink undertone to your skin look best wearing cool colors. The cool-color categories are further divided into two seasons: Winter and Summer. These two are sister seasons. They contain a range of shades that work to complement each other.

Winters look best in clear tones and dramatic contrasts. In the wintertime, have you noticed how white snow contrasts against the dark bark of empty trees that are backed up against the clear blue sky? This is a typical scene and explains the Winter person's colors! A Winter's best colors are the true primaries: very red, lemon yellow, and sky blue. Also, black, white, gray, icy pastels, true navy, royal blue, shocking pink, emerald green, and fuchsia. Winter people should avoid browns, rusts, orange, and other spicy earth tones. Winter skin tones are porcelain, snowy cream, rose beige, light to dark olive, and black. Winter hair colors are light to dark brown, charcoal, reddish black, blue-black, or white. Their eyes are deep blue, dark brown, or gray-green (*See* Figure 9-2 in the color section.)

Summer colors have the same undertones as Winter, but with a softer touch. Less contrast and more pastels for Summer! This season is truly in full bloom! Alive tones like lavender, orchid, plum, mauve, raspberry, blue-green, soft white; cool pastels like pink, mint, and clear yellow are especially good for Summer! Summer and Winter can intermix colors and still be enhancing to the cool skin tone. It's when you get into warm seasons that your skin appears dull rather than dynamic! Summer skin tones are fair, pink, pale beige, rose-toned beige, and light olive. Hair colors are light to dark brown, ash blonde, or gray. Eye colors are gray-blue, gray-green, aqua, or soft hazel. (*See* Figure 9-3 in the color section.)

Warm colors are worn by people with golden yellow undertones to their skin. It makes sense, then, that warm colors are colors with a yellow-gold cast to them. If you mixed yellow paint to the primary colors you would create the warm season's color palette. Spring and Autumn are sister seasons in the warm category.

Spring's palette of clean, fresh, warm tones would include colors such as peach, apricot, coral, orange-red, ivory, camel, medium brown, warm or yellowed navy, purple, aqua, kelly green, and warm turquoise. Spring's skin tones are creamy ivory, peach beige, and warm beige. Hair colors are light to dark blonde, strawberry blonde, golden brown, or copper. Eye colors are blue-green, topaz, aqua, golden brown, golden green, or hazel. (*See* Figure 9-4 in the color section.)

Autumn is the most vivid season. Leaves are turning bright orange, deep rust, shades of browns and yellows. These underlying tones make up the Autumn color palette. The best tones for Autumn people begin with the spicy earth tones—a full range of browns, nutmeg, rust, cinnamon, burnt orange, bronze, terra-cotta, olive, army green, teal blue, deep periwinkle, beige, camel, salmon, tomato red, and pumpkin. Autumn's skin tones are golden, ivory, peach, warm beige, and copper cast. The range of hair colors for this season is brunette with gold or red highlights, golden blonde, red, and auburn. Eye colors are dark brown, golden green, hazel, or turquoise. Autumn's undertones are the same as her sister season, Spring, yet Autumn's colors are more intense. (*See* Figure 9-5 in the color section.)

Any Color, Accurate Shade

Did you notice that some very similar colors were mentioned under different seasons? This may seem contradictory, but it's not. The key to this whole color theory and making it work is this: You can wear any color. You just need to wear the correct shade and intensity of that color for your skin tone! If an Autumn person says she can't wear yellow, she is wrong. It just has to be a golden yellow, whereas Summer's yellow is a clear lemon yellow. Using green as an example, see how the shade and intensity varies for each season. Winter's green is deep emerald; Summer's green is clear blue-green; Spring's green is a clear yellow-green; Autumn's green is olive. (*See* Figure 9-6 in the color section.) All of the seasons can wear green in their own special shade. This is a very important key to remember.

Now, staying with colors within your season is great. I just hope you won't feel restricted to those colors only. Expand into your sister season, staying within your undertone range of cool or warm.

Identifying Your Season

Now let's talk about what season you are. The most accurate way of discovering your coloring is to have a professional color analysis, if you can afford one. Choose a qualified color consultant. Many so-called trained professionals have appeared overnight on the color scene. Some are very good, others are guessing. Find out (1) what type of training the consultant has had, (2) what lighting he or she uses (natural or nontinted bulbs are best), (3) the process she will use to determine your season (usually by fabric draping), and (4) in what form your season's colors will be given to you. Prepacked paint chips are not very accurate because they fade easily. Ready-cut fabric swatches are most common. I know one color consultant who custom selects your colors using hundreds of fabric pieces. She first determines your season and then cuts swatches off the fabrics that are the most flattering to you. This method is more personalized.

If you'd like to pinpoint your season yourself, use these guidelines.

First, stare at your skin! Study the tones that make up your unique coloring. Do you see cool rosy and pink tones in your cheeks? Are your lips naturally ruby? Perhaps you see more warm yellow tints with an ivory cast. Any freckles? Is your lip color more on the beige side? Which descriptions best fit you? From the descriptions given in the previous section, which hair and eye color characterize you?

The second way to identify your season will require a few props. Gather up a wide range of solid-colored fabrics. Shirts, scarves, towels—anything with color! Remove all of your makeup. Now sit next to a big window that is letting in floods of natural light. Place a mirror in front of you and, one at a time, drape the colored fabric over your shoulder and under your chin. Watch the effects the colors have on your skin's appearance. Cool-undertoned skins will look yellowish in warm colors. Warm seasons' undertones will look grayish in cool colors. Those that make your skin glow and your eyes sparkle are for you!

Because color affects your skin's appearance, the colors you wear next to your face and on your face itself are important. Your makeup colors, specifically your liner, eye shadow, blush, and lip color, should be from your season's range of shades.

Now for the next test. Staying where you are, enter the lipstick contest as suggested by Carole Jackson, author of the popular color book *Color Me Beautiful*. The lipstick test may give you another clue in discovering your season. Try these four lipstick colors, one at a time, and see which makes you look best. Shocking pink represents the Winter season, pastel pink represents the Summer season, peach represents the Spring season, and burnt orange represents the autumn season. The perfect color is your winning season!

If you are still unsure, try comparing your skin tones to someone else who already knows her season. How do you measure up? Lighter, darker, more ivory, more olive?

Hopefully you are now fairly sure of your season. Most important, you have a definite idea of your skin undertones—either cool or warm. For further study and complete color charts see Carole Jackson's book *Color Me Beautiful* and Joanne Wallace's books *The Working Woman* and *Dress With Style*.

Color and Your Wardrobe

Discovering your best colors can serve as a guide for weeding wrong colors out of your wardrobe. That doesn't mean throw out your whole wardrobe and buy a new one! From now on, though, select clothes in your season's array of colors. As for the clothes that are not best for you anymore, give them away or wear them with a color that is good for you. It is most important that the color surrounding your face is in your season. I have a wheat-colored blazer that I love. But wheat is not very flattering against my cool-toned skin. So I wear my ruffled high-collared clear yellow blouse with it to get the positive effects of the cool color next to my face. Then I can still make good use of my wheat blazer. You can do the same with your outfits. Maybe you'll need to purchase a blouse or scarf that will make your present wardrobe colors wearable.

Build your wardrobe around three to five colors from your season's selection. This gives you mix-and-match ability. Stock up when your color season is readily available.

Color and Your Figure

Color can be used effectively to create figure illusions. It can assist in balancing out your body proportions. Light colors, white, and pale pastels attract and reflect light. This makes the areas they are covering look larger. Darker colors, on the other hand, absorb light, causing the opposite effect. The figure looks smaller. If your shoulder and bust area is smaller than your hip width, you would wear light colors on top and darker colors below your waist. The opposite is true if your hips are smaller than your shoulder width.

The color difference does not need to be drastic for it to create the illusion of an area being larger or smaller. Wearing dark tops and light pants can look unbalanced if there is a great difference between the colors. Dark colors do not mean only black, forest green, navy, and dark brown. Medium-toned blue pants are dark enough if you also wear a white blouse. The bottom color is still darker than the top.

One other color trick that petite and larger girls will like is this: Wearing the same color from top to bottom makes the figure look taller and thinner. Give it a try and see if you like the results.

Mood, Impact, Decorating

All of us are affected by the many things color can do. Color can brighten up or dull almost anything. It can generate feelings of anger or compassion. Color can even create certain atmospheres in decorating.

Depending on how a color is used, it can represent the following:

White innocence or authority
Pale yellow trustworthiness or likability
Pink calmness, softness, tender caring
Bright yellow energy, warmth
Orange high electricity
Red excitement, power, danger
Purple power or royalty
Blue coolness and refreshing calmness
Black seriousness, elegance, dignity
Gray mildness or indifference, neutrality
Green honesty, jealousy

The list goes on, but these are the most common color effects.

Use these colors in specific situations for your benefit. Let's say you are going to present a great new idea to your cheerleading squad or English class. Show up in a bright yellow outfit rather than gray! You'll be amazed how much better your ideas will sound when you are projecting energy with the colors you are wearing.

Maybe you had a dispute with your mom and the time has come to smooth the waters! Wearing red may rouse her defenses, but mint or cool blue will calm her for your big apology! Try trustworthy yellow when applying for a new job. Soft pink would be great for visiting your sick friend. See how color works to create moods and make specific impressions.

When you are redecorating your room, keep these principles in mind: First, surround yourself with a color that fits your personality. Second, find a color that says what you want to hear! Third, choose the shade of that color from your season's selection of hues.

Warmth and coolness can work in decorating. Suppose your bedroom is ice-cold most of the time. Warm it up with yellow, oranges, peaches and cream. Room too warm? Paint it sky blue or icy mint. Sounds wild, but it works!

Color and the Color Wheel

Everyone has had to make a color wheel at one time or another, maybe in art class or home economics. That same wheel will help you learn specific techniques in using color to make dynamic statements with your wardrobe.

Looking at a basic color wheel (*See* Figure 9-7 in the color section), we see the primary colors: red, yellow, and blue. These colors serve as the foundation for the rest of the colors on the wheel. Mixing the primary colors together creates the secondary colors, which are orange, green, and violet. Mixing the primaries with the secondary colors creates the tertiary colors: red-orange, yellow-orange, yellow-green, blue-green, blue-violet, and red-violet. From these and hundreds of shades in between, we get a full and complete range of colors.

Let's study the various effects of colors on each other by separating the color wheel into the major color schemes.

An *analogous* color scheme describes colors that are side by side on the color wheel. (*See* Figure 9-8 in the color section.) Violet, blue-violet, and blue are an analogous scheme. Red-orange, orange, and yellow-orange are also analogous. These tones mix well with each other because they are, in fact, mixtures of each other. They can be worn together very effectively.

Complementary color schemes are always opposite each other on the color wheel. (*See* Figure 9-9 in the color section.) Red and green, blue and orange, red-orange and blue-green, yellow-orange and blue-violet, and my favorite combination, yellow and violet. Complementary schemes are often called "contrasting schemes" because they are opposites. Also, against one another the two colors cause each other to stand out. They highlight or complement each other. This works great on the days you feel like dressing bright and bold. Split and double-complementary schemes work the same way.

Complementary schemes also work for making your eyes more noticeable. I have green eyes, so when I wear reds, my eyes are more noticeable and look even greener than they really are! Many people with blue eyes insist that wearing blue makes their eyes brighter. Just the opposite is true. Wearing complementary yellow-reds will make your eyes dance! Now perhaps you can better understand why I suggest not wearing blue-green and violet eye shadows, especially when your eyes are these colors!

A related color scheme that we can apply to our clothes is called *monochromatic*. This scheme involves one color and its various values. (*See* Figure 9-10 in the color section.) Values are created by adding white to a color. For instance, red, rose, and pink are a monochromatic scheme. Another example would be navy, true blue, and powder blue. Burnt orange, apricot, and peach or emerald green, true green, and icy green are also examples.

Lights and darks of the same color make up the monochromatic color scheme. This is the easiest scheme to use in clothing. I use it constantly in my dressing. I absolutely use it in my makeup. Monochromatic plums, roses, and pinks on my cool-toned skin make for the most together and natural makeup look. When you are experimenting with these three color schemes, remember to stay within your cool or warm color range.

Color has the ability to add so much to your appearance. It is also fun to experiment with. Discover what color combinations are best for you. Then use these colors to add a splash of brightness to your wardrobe, your mood, and your world. Wear your colors in fullest confidence that you look dazzling in them.

DAZZLE YOURSELF WITH COLOR

Project Page

1. Discover your own unique coloring. Follow the instructions that begin on page 149. Record the results of each test here. See the season descriptions to answer this first question.
    a. *Skin Tone*   *Hair Color*   *Eye Color*
    _____
    _____
    _____
    _____

    b. Using solid-colored fabrics, which colors enhance your skin's appearance?_____

    Which colors appear to drain color from your skin?_____
    _____
    _____

    c. The lipstick test: Which color looks best on you?
    _____ shocking pink (Winter)
    _____ pastel pink (Summer)
    _____ peach (Spring)
    _____ burnt orange (Autumn)

    d. Compare your skin tone to someone else's. Are you
    _____ lighter   _____ more ivory   _____ more pink
    _____ darker   _____ more olive   _____ more yellow

2. Turn to the color wheel. Find your favorite color, then look directly across from it to see what the complementary color is. Put an outfit together using those colors.

3. Choose an analogous color scheme that attracts your eye. Use these colors to create a new look for yourself.

4. Now try monochromatic dressing. Remember, that's light and dark hues of one color.

5. One-color dressing usually creates a classic and conservative, neat and tidy, pulled-together look. Choose one color and dress yourself in it from head to toe!

6. What colors have you decorated your environment with? What do these colors say—bright and energetic or mild and calm?

   _____
   _____
   _____

7. Choose three to five colors in your season's colors to build a mix-and-match wardrobe.

10 FUNCTIONING FASHION
A Wardrobe That Works

Bring on the fashion! Clothes, clothes, and more clothes! Can you believe the way designers come up with cuter and classier clothes every season? Isn't it true that by the time you've finally saved up enough baby-sitting money and have bought those jeans everyone is wearing, a new style with a great new look appears on the jean scene?

Fashion is like that. It changes each season and gets better every year. If only we didn't have to be money conscious. Let's see, I'd own one of everything and I must have it in every color! How about you?

Besides being lots of fun, clothing is a practical necessity. It is something we all need. I'm glad we don't live in the days of Adam and Eve—fig leaves just wouldn't do it for me, especially since I love being covered and wearing lots of layers.

Clothing is definitely a covering for your body, but it is more than that. Clothing is an outer reflection of your inner self. This isn't totally true since some of us would dress differently if we could afford to. But for the most part, what you wear and how you wear it can tell a lot about things like these:

Your age. It has always been easy to tell a teenager from her parents by the way she dresses. It's doubtful that you'd see many moms in denim miniskirts these days, but a teenager, probably so.

Your personality. Clothing expresses to others whether you are conservative, sporty, economical, jazzy, or even romantic. These are all different styles of dressing.

Economic situation. In our society, the labels you wear, the types of fabrics you choose, the stores where you shop, often classify you. Of course, this system is very unfair. The value and importance of the inner person can't be justly evaluated by the clothes she wears.

Your occupation. You can usually tell who is the cook and who is the waitress, a full-time mom or a businesswoman, a nurse or a doctor, by the clothes each of them wears.

Even though clothes are fun and decorative and more than a covering, they are not everything! Some people act as if they are, but they aren't. We often find ourselves jealous of the girl who gets to wear the latest high-quality fashions. We might feel inadequate if we aren't wearing the current look being shown all over the best magazines. It may make us feel second-class. If you ever feel this way, stop and take a second look.

The Bible is clear on many things, and clothing is one of them. Jesus tells us not to be hung up on what we wear. He says that God knows you need clothes and that He will provide you with what you *need*. How? Well, maybe He'll provide you with a job so you can earn the money.

The Bible also says not to be jealous of people who are dressed perfectly every day. A person's specialness doesn't come from what she is wearing on the outside but how she is dressed on the inside!

Magazines and department stores can help us out with new ideas, but we don't have to arrange our outfits just like store mannequins. Pick and choose what fits your personality and what you are comfortable wearing. It is more important to wear what looks good on you than it is to be dressed in the latest style.

It may be hard in your junior high and high school years to discover your clothing personality. That's okay. You have a chance to try various looks to find out what's best for you. Some people find a clothing style that fits them and they never change. Others, like myself, dress differently all their lives!

Let's begin by looking at different fashion styles and see if we can create for you a wardrobe that fits your personality and that works together to help you get the most out of every piece of clothing hanging in your closet. That's functioning fashion—having a wardrobe that works!

Styles: Classics and Fads

It would be a waste for me to fill this chapter with today's current style of dress. Fashion changes so fast that soon there will no doubt be a whole new set of designs filling the magazine pages and walking the halls at your school. So, let me at least share with you the basic information on wardrobing. *Wardrobe* just refers to the collection of goodies hanging in your closet.

Classics and fads are a good place to start. Classics are those timeless, ageless, practical styles that do not go out of fashion. (*See* Figure 10-1.) They will vary slightly from year to year in cut and color, but they are dependable. Cardigan sweaters, blazers, button-down oxford blouses, shirt dresses, pleated and A-line skirts, turtleneck and cowl neck sweaters, are all examples of classics.

Fads are those fun and flashy styles

Timeless Classic

Flashy Fad

Figure 10-1.

Figure 10-2.

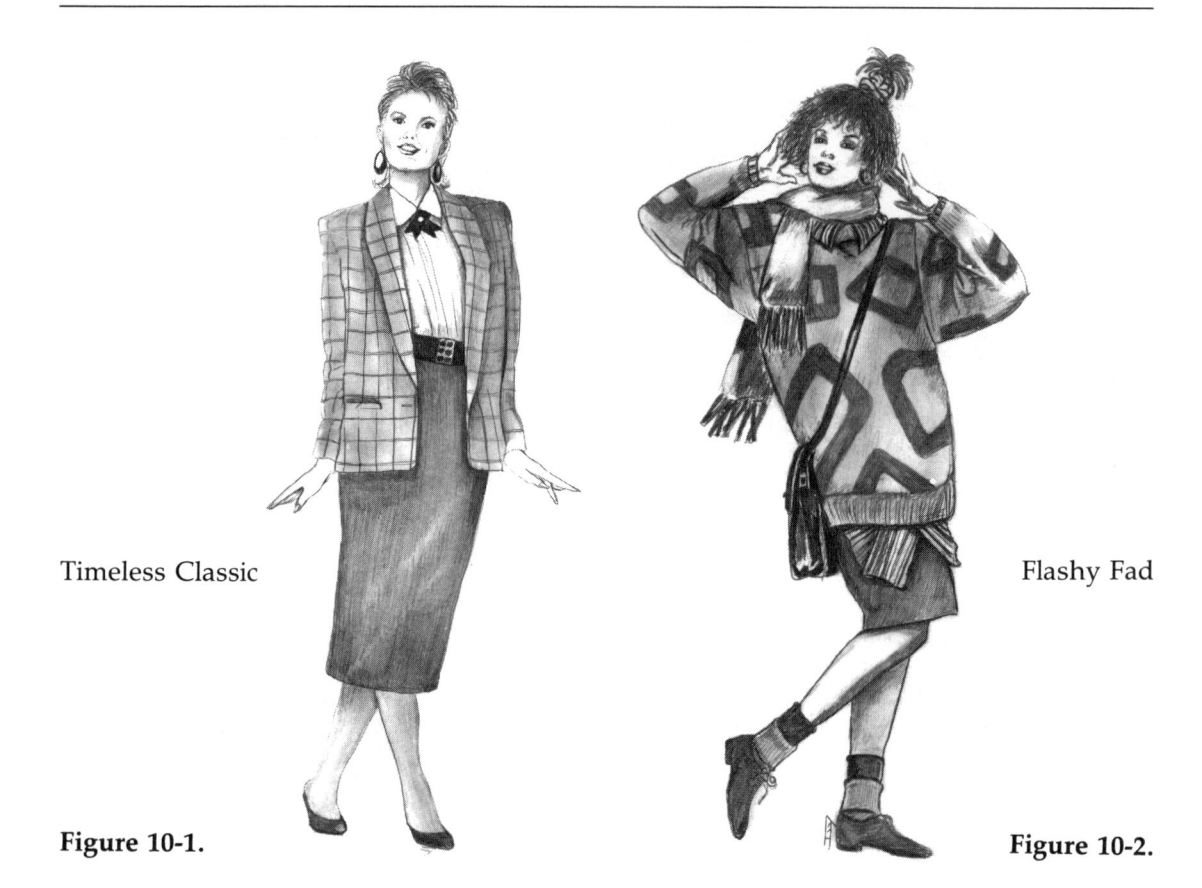

that instantly appear on the fashion scene, then disappear just as fast. (*See* Figure 10-2.) If you wear that same fad a year later, you are way behind the times! Fads need to be purchased sparingly. They are fun and add flair to your wardrobe but can be frivolous investments. Buying one or two fad garments or accessories per season should keep you well updated in your fashions. Adapt the latest designs to your figure, life-style, and personality.

Clothing and fashion are meant to be enjoyed, but don't run out and buy every new fad. Wait to see what will be out in another six months.

Classics make a better investment than fads. Use your best judgment. Remember, the goal for designers and clothing companies is to sell their merchandise! That is why each season they come up with new styles and colors.

Now, speaking of designers, become familiar with labels and designers. You will probably discover a couple of designers who continuously design according to your clothing tastes. This can make your shopping more convenient. It is also more practical because when you buy within the same few lines, you will find outfits that coordinate in color and style.

Another bonus of knowing designer brands is that you can look for well-made look-alikes for about half the cost! That's smart shopping.

Being a Smart Shopper

There is a real art to shopping. What influences your shopping? How you feel? The mood you are in? What your wardrobe is in need of? Many of us females are mood shoppers. This is a fun way to shop but can leave us with a closetful of unwearable clothes—nothing to match the color, wrong style shoes, and the list goes on!

Here are some smart shopper questions:

1. Do you shop for quality or quantity? Quantity shoppers love to buy, buy, buy. "The more clothes the better," is their motto. But really, seven $10.98 blouses in seven different colors? Quality shoppers look for well-made garments that will match a variety of pieces already in their wardrobes. They may spend a few more dollars, but their investments usually last longer. If you strive to be a quality-minded shopper but are on a limited budget, save up or put the item on layaway. There is no extra charge for this service.
2. Are you aware of color when you shop? Even though that sweater is a beautiful emerald green and only $29.98, why buy it when you have nothing in your wardrobe to match it? When you stay within a selected color range, you will have more options in your wardrobe for mix and match.
3. Do you overbuy on the same item? Let's talk jeans. I'll bet you have more than two pairs. Most kids have button-ups, tight-leg, faded, or print. At this writing, the latest is colored jeans! That adds up to too many! Skip a season and see what comes out next year! Don't overbuy on the same thing.
4. Are you crazy over the word SALE? I am. It's in my blood. My mom is a great sale shopper and garage sale goer. But—too many times I come home with my bargain outfit and never wear it. It wasn't really what I wanted, or maybe the color was a bit off. Sometimes bargain clothes aren't bargains at all. Some aren't made well. Check seams, buttons, zippers, hems, matching stripes, and topstitching. Quality counts.
5. Are you stuck in one department or do you cross-shop in all the departments? I'm sure your fingers comb their way through the Junior department first—that's natural. However, the Junior department is the trendiest department. Expand into the Misses once in a while. It often has small sizes (4–6) and more useful, classic styles.
6. Are you attracted to "Dry Clean Only" labels? They are usually attached to very pretty fabrics. You'll wind up spending a lot more on the garment than the sticker price if it can't handle at-home cleaning.
7. Finally, are you intimidated by pushy salesclerks? The decision to buy a garment is yours and yours alone. You're the one who is going to wear it, not her! And not your friends! Group shopping is great for Saturday afternoons. You probably check out more sights than just clothes. But you will be able to accomplish more serious shopping by yourself or with one other person who can be helpful.

Being a smart shopper is an art worth developing. Proverbs 31:14 and 16 refer to a woman who is a smart shopper. Verse 14 says this type of woman searches out good buys; she brings food or products from far away. Verse 16 says she considers a field and buys it. This smart woman does not buy on the spur of the moment. No impulse purchases for her. She considers the value, worth, practicality, and appropriateness of the garment before she spends her well-earned money on it. She is a smart shopper who asks herself, "Why do I want this? Why should or shouldn't I buy this?" Smart questions. The Lord wants you to be a good manager of your money. Don't blow your bucks on careless decisions. Be a smart shopper!

Dressing Your Figure

Part of being an intelligent shopper is knowing what you are looking for when you shop. What looks good on you? What lines enhance your appearance? Which styles are best for dressing your figure? Do the fabrics you select really matter? Let's investigate....

Use of Line

Lines created by stripes, seams, pleats, detailed designs, or even a row of buttons are a tool in achieving your desired look. Horizontal lines add width. Vertical lines add an illusion of height and slenderness. Curved lines on collars, ruffles, or seams add fullness and softness. Diagonal lines add height and minimize size. All of these are illusions. You don't actually become taller or wider or slimmer! Nonetheless, using line creatively can help you dress to enhance your figure. (*See* Figures 10-3, 10-4, 10-5, 10-6.)

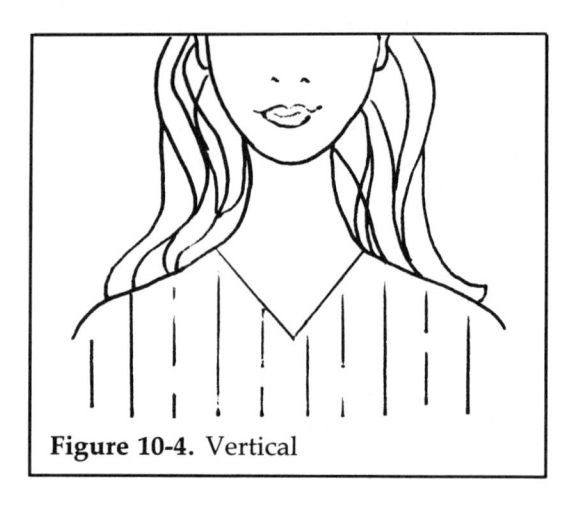

Figure 10-4. Vertical

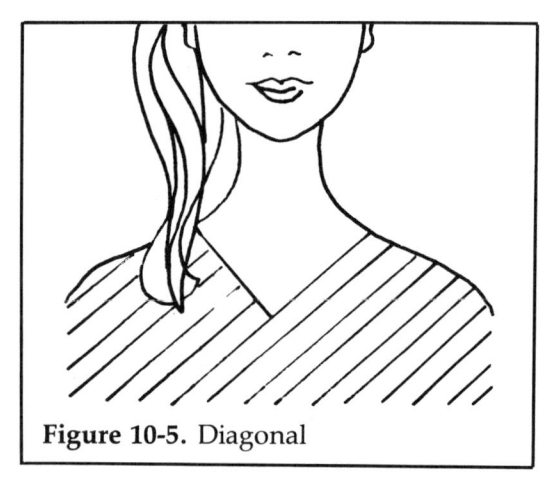

Figure 10-5. Diagonal

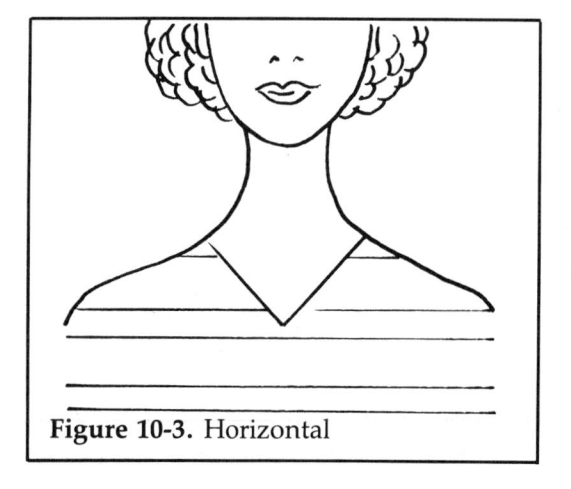

Figure 10-3. Horizontal

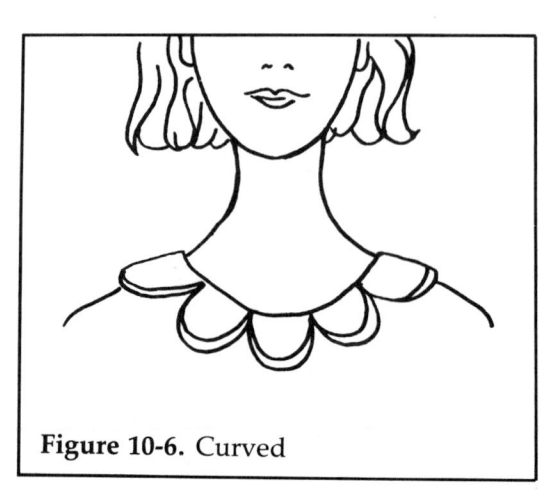

Figure 10-6. Curved

Use of Style

The cut and style of a garment can affect your figure's appearance. Knowing your figure type will help you dress it into proportion. Remember, there is no perfect figure since we are all made individually. There are no two people alike and no such thing as a right or wrong figure type. However, there is a sense of balance and proportion that you can achieve in your dressing. The following are simply suggestions in using clothing to balance your features.

The Hourglass Figure. This figure type is fairly close to being evenly proportioned. Make adjustments where needed when necessary.

The Inverted Triangle. This figure type has a larger bosom or shoulders with slender hips. You need emphasis below the waist to balance your upper proportions. Try gathered or pleated pants and skirts. Wear plain-cut, non-puffed, and no-front-pocket blouses or shirts. Avoid wide belts and horizontal lines. You need your necklace to hang above or below your bustline to avoid added fullness in that area.

The Triangle. This figure type is exactly opposite the last one. Your smaller bosom or shoulders and full hips are best dressed with emphasis above your waistline. Try tops with front pockets, ruffles, pleats, horizontal stripes, puffed sleeves, and padded shoulders. No, not all at the same time! You can easily wear the layered look—blouses under sweaters or double-breasted jackets over a sweater vest and blouse. A-line skirts are better on you than straight tube-type styles. Avoid gathered pants and skirts. Choose soft fabrics rather than crisp or bulky ones.

The Round Figure. You are curvy above and below the waist area. You will do best avoiding overemphasis in the bust or hip area. Tight clothes or frilly designs are not for you. Straight tops, dresses, or jackets with nonfitted waists are great. Don't wear belts or gathers at your tummy. Beware of tops that end right on the curviest part of your hip. They will make you appear wider because of the horizontal line they create. Try to be conservative.

The Square Figure. This figure type is usually short-waisted, with shoulder and hip area about the same width. Wide belts and fitted waists may not work for you. Avoid shoulder pads that may make your figure appear boxy. Gathers will soften your hip area.

The Petite Figure. You are usually under five feet, three inches tall and can take any of the previous forms. You are special, though, because you get your own section in many department stores! Wear vertical designs and outfits that are the same color from head to toe. This makes you appear taller—assuming you want to look taller, that is. Avoid long skirts, tops, and blazers. Pullover sweaters should end at the top of your hipbone, not near your lower hip. Long tops will visually cut your figure in half, making you look dwarfed. No chunky jewelry. Wear accessories in proportion with your size.

The Tall Figure. You are, on an average, five feet, eight inches tall. Solid colors head to toe are not a requirement for you. Longer tops and jackets are easier for you to wear. Avoid crop tops and skirts or pants that make you look as if you are all leg. Skirts that look best on you will be at least mid-calf or longer, not knee-length. It is easier for your figure type to pull off high-fashion dressing. Cuffs on pants minimize long legs.

Short-Waisted Figures. You have less distance from your shoulders to your waist. To make this area look longer wear belts that match the color of what you're wearing above your waist rather than below it. This applies, of course, to when you are tucking your top in. You can also wear tops and sweaters that rest near the top of your hip, making your torso appear longer.

Long-Waisted Figures. You look good in fitted clothes, but can appear out of proportion if you aren't careful. When you wear your tops tucked in, wear belts that match the color of your pants or skirt. This makes the waistline look higher and your waist shorter.

Necks. Long necks should try medium-length hair, lots of scarves, turtle and cowl necks, and turned-up collars. No deep V necks for you. Short necks want the V shape to make the neck area look longer. Stand-up collars and turtlenecks won't be your best friend. Short hair is said to be most flattering on you.

Calves. A quick hint for thin and thick calves. Thin legs are complemented by narrow skirts. Flared skirts will make thin legs look like sticks. Just the opposite is true for thick calves. Avoid the fitted skirt and go for the fuller-cut styles. The length of your skirt is best below the widest part of your calf. Straight-leg pants will look better on you than pegged styles.

Faces. To best complement your face shape, do not repeat the shape of your jawline in the neckline of your garment. For instance, a square jaw is softened if it is surrounded by a curved neckline. The rounded face is best with a V neck or square neckline.

Remember, these are only guidelines, not absolutes. Use them to create balance. You can't possibly wear the same cuts and styles all the time. That could make dressing boring and dull.

Fabrics Affect Your Figure, Too

The fabric you choose can make or break your outfit and figure. As a general rule, heavier fabrics, nubby knits, and stiff textures add visual weight to your figure. So do shiny-surfaced fabrics because they reflect light. Smooth, soft-fitting fabrics with dull or matte finishes will not add the visual weight.

As I mentioned, matching solid tones worn head to toe can make your figure look tall and slimmer. Prints and plaids have a definite effect as well. They usually either add visual weight or have an effect on height. It depends on the design. One point to remember, since we are talking about proportions: Wear prints and plaids that are the same-size scale as your figure. Tiny figures that wear large prints look overwhelmed. So it goes for larger figures that choose tiny prints. Choose those that best fit your body size.

This same principle applies to your accessories—jewelry, belts, scarves, and purses. Select accessories proportionate to your body size.

Organizing Your Wardrobe

If you are like most other teens, your clothes are jammed into your closet, some hanging half off the hanger, some inside out, others buttoned wrong, and several in desperate need of an iron or laundry basket. I wouldn't doubt that many of you even have clothes on doorknobs, bedposts, over chairs, or—the worst—on the floor!

Most of us have too many clothes. Yet, each morning we stand in front of the closet for what seems like hours because we can't find anything to wear! The problem is we have not planned our wardrobe. Here is your chance to get organized and have more outfits than you have occasions to wear them.

First, unclutter your closet. Get out all the things you have not worn in the last year. Allow your wardrobe some breathing space. Ask yourself why you haven't worn these garments—they don't fit, they are out of style, need repairs, are worn and tattered looking, or you just have nothing to go with them.

Take your pile of "don't wears" and drop them off at your church's clothing drive or your local thrift shop. I usually try to find someone who can make good use of my "don't wear" clothes. I also try to stick to my personal fair-exchange policy. If I want a new dress, I give one away. If I need new slacks, I find someone who can wear the ones that don't fit me anymore. It makes it so much fun to give things away. Then I don't feel as if I've wasted those other purchases, and at the same time I'm weeding out the optional clothes, leaving myself with a wardrobe that is more workable.

Second, make a pile of "need repairs." A missing button can put your favorite blouse or dress out of order! That is silly. If you can't find the original button, go buy a complete new set for the garment. Buttons, zippers, snaps, and thread for hems are not expensive! Fixing your repair pile will give you more to wear. Don't delay—do it today!

Next, separate your clothes into the two major times of year: spring/summer and fall/winter. If you live in a warm climate year round as I do, just keep your cool-weather clothes in the back of your closet for easy access on those chilly evenings. Put the clothes you are not presently wearing in a garment bag or cover them with a clean plastic bag (with the exception of leather, suede, and furs, as this damages them). When the seasons begin to change and you uncover your sleeping beauties, you'll feel as if you have a new wardrobe. The effect is not the same if you have been staring at the same clothes all year round. One note—when storing wools and sweaters, use mothballs in drawers and bags. Keep the mothballs or flakes from touching your garments.

Grouping Your Garments

Now you are ready to group your clothes according to type: blouses, shirts (including active wear T-shirts and sweat shirts), jackets, jeans, pants, shorts, skirts, dresses, and sweaters. Arrange them from light shades to dark shades. I go one step further with my blouses, separating short-sleeved from long-sleeved. Now you have a clear view of your wardrobe. Do you like what you see? Is it a true reflection of you? Does it seem there are some missing pieces to your wardrobe puzzle?

Piecing the Puzzle Together

Dressing is not meant to be a hit-or-miss maze, though at times it can be puzzling. Now is the time to make the pieces fit together by discovering what pieces of the puzzle are not there. Start by looking at the clues!

Let's say you have several tops with navy blue in them—one is a solid, one a print, one a plaid—but you don't have a navy skirt or pants. That's one missing piece! Adding one pair of pants in the right color can give you several new options in your wardrobe.

Another clue: Perhaps you have too many prints or plaids. This really limits your wardrobe. You can't wear a print blouse with a print skirt unless they came together. To get more flexibility from your clothes, decide to purchase either your tops or bottoms mostly in solids. Solids mix and match much easier. If you are starting over with your wardrobe, I strongly suggest concentrating on buying solids. Basic colors which go well with other colors are navy, gray, black, white, cream, and natural. These are best for pants or skirts.

Choose three to five colors from your color category that blend together well, and purchase within that range. For instance, the cool category could consist of navy, white, pink, gray, and black. These colors and the various shades of each will intermix well. The warm-category girl can begin with peach, ivory, cinnamon brown, rust, and coral. You will find you can coordinate more outfits by sticking with a particular color theme. Add other colors later, or buy inexpensive accessories such as belts, scarves, or jewelry.

The next clue to finding those missing puzzle pieces is style. Do you have the latest fads from each season but no classics? Building a wardrobe means using classics to lay your foundation and fashionable fads for added dimensions only!

What about fabrics? A cotton T-shirt, silk blouse, wool sweater vest, and polyester skirt don't work well together. Build with casual or semi-dressy fabrics, then expand with special fabrics along the way.

Now, make a list of the items you discovered you need. Put the items in order of priority and take your list with you when you shop. Stick to your needs. Don't go out shopping for a cream crew-neck sweater and return home with another red one. Complete the puzzle first!

The Completed Puzzle

The reason we have been looking for missing puzzle pieces is so you can create a complete wardrobe. This is your goal in building a workable wardrobe. This includes making individual outfits complete as well, with belts, nylons, scarves, shoes, and all the trimmings. Colored nylons add a finishing touch to dresses and skirts. Try knee-highs under pants or long skirts.

Shoes should be well cared for on a rack, in a shoe bag, or neatly lined up on your closet floor. Keep them clean and polished. Basic colors will give you the most flexibility. You probably need only one or two pairs of pumps for dressing up. Beige or neutral is best. Flats and sport shoes are more practical for school. Choose colors that you can wear with almost any outfit. Your shoe color should not be brighter than the color of the outfit you are wearing. In fact, if it is the same color as your pants, dress, or skirt, it will make your legs look long and more slender. Many of the creative syles of shoes these days make them an accessory as well as a necessity.

The chart included here is meant to help in your organizing and building process. Fill out the chart for your spring/summer and fall/winter clothes.

Wardrobe Chart

For each category briefly describe each garment and what you have and/or need to coordinate with it. Designate whether the chart is for your casual or dressy clothes and for your spring/summer or fall/winter wardrobe.

GARMENTS		ITEMS TO COORDINATE			
CASUAL or DRESSY	SPRING/SUMMER or FALL/WINTER	SHOES BOOTS NYLONS	JEWELRY	BELTS SCARVES	PURSES	NEED
TOPS:						
BLOUSES:						
PANTS/JEANS:						
SKIRTS:						
SWEATERS:						
SWEAT SUITS:						
DRESSES:						
JACKETS/COATS:						
OTHER:						

Watch how your wardrobe comes alive as you discover new combinations and purchase pieces needed to complete your individual wardrobe puzzle.

Basic Survival Wardrobe for Teens

Every girl is different, and dressing styles are different in every part of the United States. I found that out when I moved from Oklahoma to California. But nonetheless, I have put together a basic survival wardrobe as a guideline for those of you who feel at a loss. These basic tools in your survival kit should give you a well-rounded wardrobe that is ready for every occasion.

One Casual Dress. A solid-colored dress that can be accessorized sporty or semi-dressy is a must in every closet! Keep it fairly plain and classic in style.

One Skirt. A calf-length skirt in a versatile fabric such as cotton or denim would give you the most options. Select a reasonable color. Denim miniskirts are popular but should not be the only style skirt you own.

Two Pairs of Jeans. If you are like most of the girls I know, jeans are the main article in your wardrobe. Two pairs is practical. Choose two different styles—one for school, one for other occasions. Avoid making both of them faded. For example, I have casual and dress jeans.

One Dressy Pant. Church meetings, dinner out, dates—they all call for something other than jeans! Try a cotton polyester blend or a linen fabric for a great-looking pair of dress pants. Side and back opening styles have a dressier look than a front zipper.

One Dressy Blouse. Silky-feel blouses are not part of a teen's everyday wardrobe, but it is a good idea to have a dressy blouse for special occasions. White or cream gives the most versatility. Add a gold or silver necklace or a strand of pearls.

Two Casual Blouses. One classic oxford cloth in a button-down or Peter Pan collar plus one cotton casual blouse are great for starters. These can easily be worn under a sweater, dress, or over your dress and belted.

One Sweater. This is nearly impossible for me! I love sweaters. It's a good thing, too, because I'm cold most of the time. A basic crew neck is a good foundation for your sweater collection.

Jackets. Most teens don't wear blazers, but I would suggest a cardigan that you can wear open, buttoned, or belted. It looks more like a part of your outfit than a coat does.

One Sweat Suit. I can't imagine a wardrobe without a sweat suit. Get tops and pants to match and in a color that works well with the three to five colors you have chosen to begin your wardrobe with. Sweat-shirt dressing has become a great compromise for dressing up but feeling comfortable.

Decorative sweats help make dressing easy.

Shoes. Your basic shoe starting kit can include one of each basic style: flat, sandal, heel, and tennis shoe. Choose neutral tones such as beige, cream, or gray to match a wide variety of clothing colors. For further shoe suggestions *see* "Fancy Footwear."

You will probably have more clothes and shoes than these. This list is meant to be a guide—a foundation for you to build upon. Keep in mind that your goal is to have a coordinated wardrobe that allows you to mix and match effectively.

FUNCTIONING FASHION

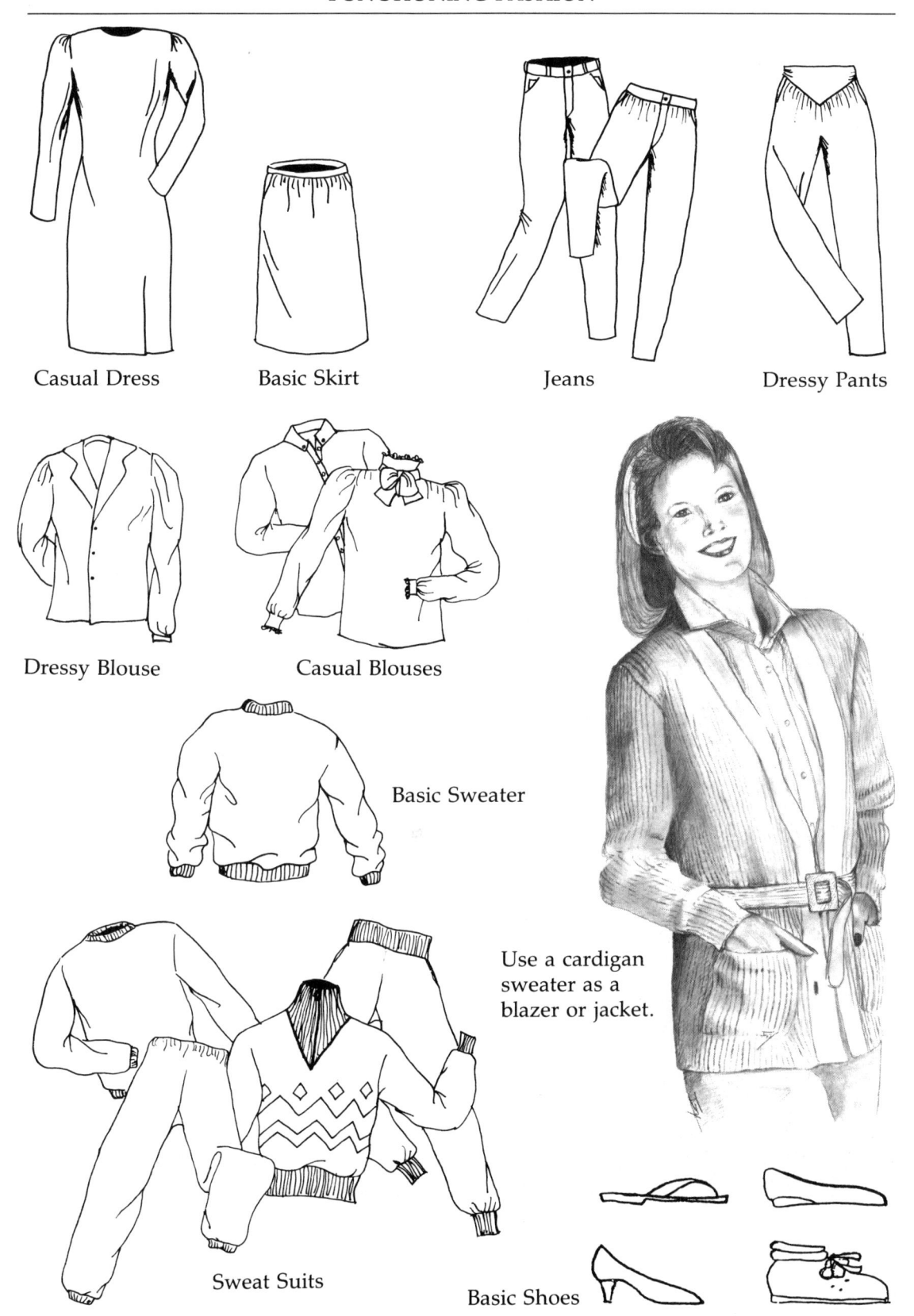

Casual Dress　　Basic Skirt　　Jeans　　Dressy Pants

Dressy Blouse　　Casual Blouses

Basic Sweater

Use a cardigan sweater as a blazer or jacket.

Sweat Suits　　Basic Shoes

Accessories—an Additional Touch

The best way to brighten your wardrobe and add creative complements is through accessories. Jewelry, belts, scarves, purses, bags, socks, sunglasses, nylons—the list goes on and on. Accessories can bring instant life and fashion to your wardrobe without breaking your budget. (*See* Figures 10-7, 10-8.)

As a general rule, accessories should be worn in proportion to your body size. If you are making a particular statement with a big bag or earrings or such, then your accessories may not be the same scale as the rest of you. Some outfits demand specific accessories, though staying close to your body size is best.

Jewelry

Jewelry has always been fun for me. I love to wear it. Today's jewelry manufacturers have made it possible to have fine-looking jewelry at fine prices! The only real jewelry I own is my wedding ring and a ring my parents gave me on my twenty-first birthday. The rest is either 14 karat gold-filled, sterling silver plated, or color costume jewelry. I learned in my early modeling days to never carry real jewelry with me on modeling jobs or interviews, so I've never purchased expensive pieces.

Well-made costume jewelry allows me more variety on a conservative budget. I have colored earrings and bracelets to match the main colors in my wardrobe: white, pink, navy, black, and red. You don't have to spend a lot of money on these. Ten to twelve dollars is the average cost of earrings and bracelets. (*See* Figure 10-9.)

Pierced earrings are easier to find than clip-ons. I don't have pierced ears, so I am very aware of this. Surgical steel posts or gold posts are better for most ears. Infected pierced ears are no fun! If you fall in love with a pair of pierced earrings but don't have pierced ears, try earring converters. Converters are clip-on attachments that make most pierced earrings wearable for those of us who don't have extra holes in our ears.

For an unusual twist in your bracelets, try bracelet-style watches. They double as bracelets beautifully. Watches have become popular acces-

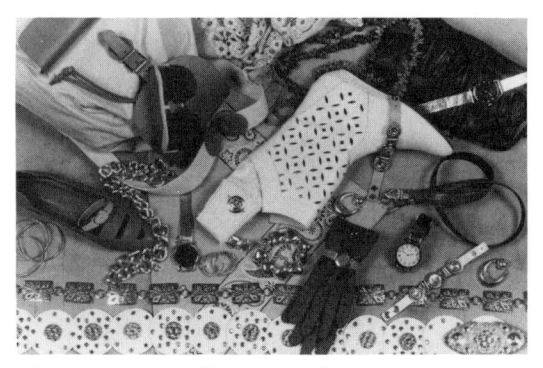

Figure 10-7. Fun watches, sunglasses, bracelets, belts, bags, and more! Spruce up your daytime wardrobe with sporty accessories.

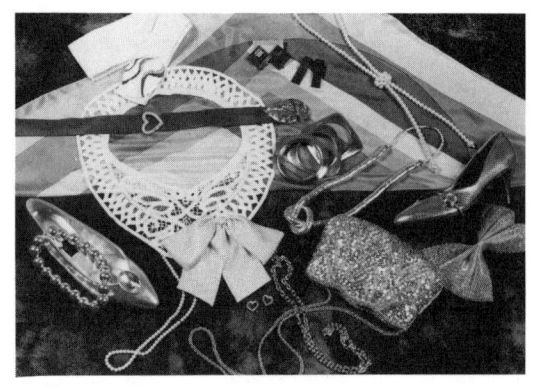

Figure 10-8. Rhinestones, sequins, lace, and pearls! Your special-occasion wardrobe will be enhanced with dressy accessories.

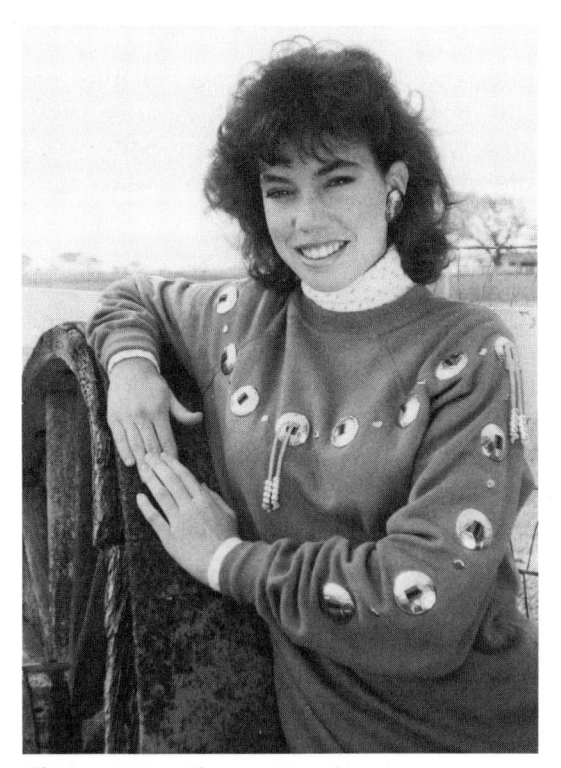

Figure 10-9. This sweat shirt with decorative conchos and matching concho earrings gives Jenni a fun yet neat appearance, using costume jewelry.

sories. Decorative watches have become a must, and you can find them everywhere. I have even seen two or three watches being worn together. You are sure to be on time that way!

Along with my colored jewelry, I have a variety of gold and silver tones. According to color-analysis systems, gold jewelry is for warm-undertoned skins and silver is for cool-undertoned skins. I have always worn gold tones and disregarded this theory. However, since silver jewelry is the craze right now, and I'm currently managing an accessory boutique, I have tried silver and must confess: I love it! It really does look better against my skin than I had imagined it would. So, I wear both, but I don't mix them. If you buy a piece of jewelry that mixes silver and gold tones—okay. But don't wear a gold chain with silver earrings and a colored bracelet. It doesn't work. Matched sets or at least matched tones give a more together look. (*See* Figure 10-10.)

Unusually fashioned pieces of jewelry are great, but buy wisely. It's no fun to have an expensive necklace stashed away in your jewelry box because it's no longer the thing to wear.

Real jewelry is often bought as an investment. It is definitely longer lasting. The gold and silver market dictates the cost of fine jewelry. The same is true for beautiful precious, semi-

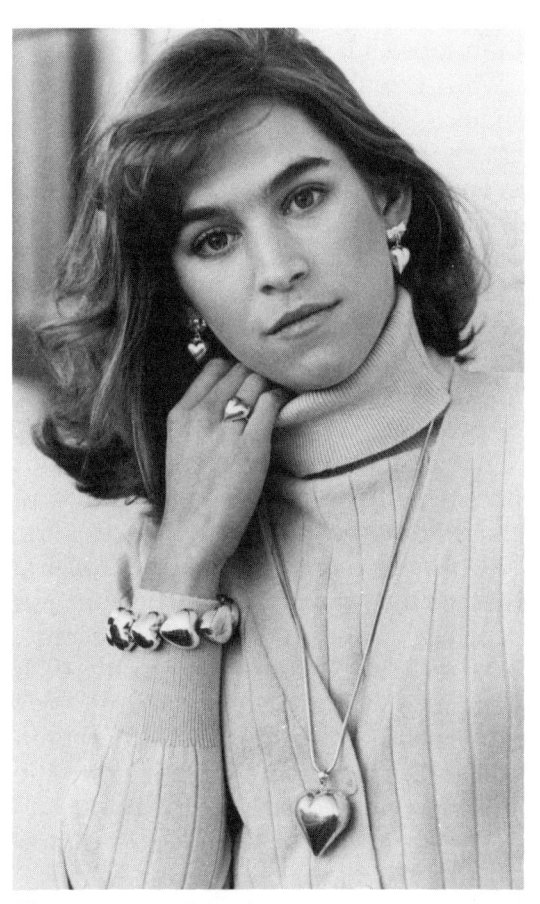

Figure 10-10. Match your jewelry to get a real "together" look. Using all silver tones in matching hearts gives this a more styled appearance for Sally.

precious, and gem stones. Their value is determined by their durability and availability. There are gorgeous designs these days. However, I doubt that expensive jewelry is practical for most teens.

Pearls are a classic item and their versatility is great. Whether you go dressy or casual, pearls are ready to go with you. Ivory or white pearls are most popular. Colored strands are terrific, too. Invest in a matching earring-and-necklace set. Choose your favorite type: cultured or freshwater. Imitation pearls can look as good as the real thing. Select a strand with glass beads rather than plastic, hand-tied rather than loose strung.

Glitz is really in: crystal, rhinestones, sequins, glass. Match it to your outfit. In the past, sparkle was kept for evening wear or special occasions only. Today it is brought into everyday dressing. Try it. If it feels as if you're playing make-believe, it's not for you.

Pins are loads of fun and can add a touch of decoration to any outfit. Place them on lapels, collars, hats, jackets, or pockets.

Before we move on, one note about necklaces. The necklace length and shape should complement the neckline of your garment. Necklaces crossing the neckline make it look choppy. For boat-neck and crew-neck designs, wear a short choker-type necklace. If you are wearing a blouse or cowl neck underneath the other neckline, then you are not necessarily restricted to the choker-style necklace.

Belts

You can find a huge selection of styles: wide, thin, elastic, cloth, buckle, wrap, waist, or hip rest. Belts are a standard accessory that never goes out of style. Select a belt that fits the mood of your outfit. A satin jump suit with a woven cotton belt won't blend.

Purses

Big ones, small ones, in-between ones—I have them all. And in every color! Well, not in *every* color. Purses and bags are more than purposeful for transporting your daily necessities; they also complete your outfit. Purses that match your clothing with their color and style will give you a real together look. Here again, because I want variety, I get the best purse I can find at the lowest price. Vinyl fabrics are good for me. They can get wet, be wiped off, polished, even folded! Some ladies swear by leather. Yes, leather has that smart look and is long lasting, but it isn't practical or priced right for the wear and tear some of us put on our bags. (*See* "Visual Graces" on page 41 for fabric, color, and carrying tips.)

Nylons

Colored nylons were a wonderful invention. Match tones to your dress, skirt, or pants. Lighter shades are best. Dark shades can look heavy unless they are worn with a solid-colored skirt and are the same color as the skirt. Choose sheer rather than opaque. Wear colored knee-highs with pants. Hopefully your colored nylons will be the same color as your shoes, though cream and white nylons can be worn with almost any color shoe. If they do not match, your leg may look chopped up. Choosing a neutral shade, one close to your skin tone, will always look good.

Textured nylons are nice as long as they do not fight a print or plaid in the fabric of your clothing. Control-top and light-support nylons are great for those of us who like the tight-fitting style. Cotton-crotch styles can take the place of underpants but should be laundered after each wearing. You can hand wash your nylons regularly. This restores their shape and prolongs the beginning of most runs. I'm sure you know the nail polish trick. If your nylon begins to run, stop it with nail polish. Clear polish, that is! Of course if the run can be seen, toss the nylons and buy a new pair.

Socks

Socks are perfect for casual dressing. Knee-highs, mid-calf, anklets, wool, cotton, or nylon. Take your pick! Socks are fun for adding color—perhaps repeating a color from your blouse or sweater. This pulls the outfit together. Decorative socks with polka dots, stripes, bows, even appliqués, add a sense of style and impression to your outfit. My sister-in-law gave me a pair of *real* creative socks for my birthday: aqua toes and heels, lavender foot and band around the top, with a black-and-white-checked ankle as a background for a sewn-on leather cat wearing a fuchsia bow around his neck. He even has whiskers made from yarn. Now that's decorative!

Fancy Footwear

There is such a wide variety of shoes available in style, design, and color. Some are just for fun, others are a necessity.

The first shoe you'll need is a flat. This means little or no heel. Flats are worn with casual and semi-dressy clothes. Choose a neutral tone like beige, cream, or gray, or a tone that blends with the majority of colors in your wardrobe. Wearing pants or skirts, nylons, and shoes all the same color will make your legs look longer and your outfit more classic.

For those dressier occasions, a pump shoe with a medium high heel is just what you'll need. Again, choose a neutral tone to allow yourself versatility. Wearing heels is a matter of personal preference. If you don't care for a high heel, try a one-and-a-half-inch heel. This will give you a dressier feel. It also gives a more graceful look to your legs and walk. Stay away from ankle-strap styles. They'll make your legs look short and choppy.

Sandals are great foot savers for the summertime. Choose the style you like the best: thongs, slip-ons, heel strap with a side buckle, or even tie-ons!

Every wardrobe needs a pair or two of tennis shoes. As for color, white goes with almost everything. Padded high tops give extra support, but the more fitted, less-bulky style gives a sleeker look. Tennis shoes have gained a new following since sweat-shirt dressing has become so popular. They are comfortable, casual, and they put pep in your step!

Boots continue to be a featured item in foot fashions. Knee-high, mid-calf, and ankle boots all have their own look. They are super with skirts, pants, or jeans. Choose from a dress boot with a heel, a cowboy boot, or a contemporary cut with a flat heel.

When selecting footwear, proper fit is as important as fashion. A good-fitting shoe will complement your posture, your walk, and will keep your feet and legs from aching. Check for comfortable toe space, proper arch, and a hugging heel. Your feet will feel better and so will you!

Sunglasses

Another practical necessity that has become an accessory is sunglasses. Choose a style that complements your face shape, personality, and wardrobe. The darker the lenses the more protective they are to your eyes.

Sunglasses can also be used as a headband. This is one of my fastest and easiest hair tricks!

Scarves

There is so much you can do with a simple scarf. It can accent your outfit by adding color, design, and dimension. Wear it around your neck, in your hair, or as a belt. Scarves can fill in a neckline or cover it up. Coordinate your scarf color with your outfit and with the fabric of your outfit. A wool scarf with a T-shirt dress will look odd. So will a silk scarf on a cotton blouse. Keep casual fabrics together and dressy fabrics together.

Ready-made pin-on bows are great looking and save you the hassle of tying that bow just right. When correctly attached, pin-on bows can double as hair bows on ponytails.

Like scarves, lace collars can add softness, romance, and feminine frill to your blouses, sweaters, and dresses. When you attach the lace collar, get it as even with the neckline of your garment as possible.

Here are a few scarf-tying ideas. Various scarf sizes and shapes allow you to create a variety of styles. Don't be shy, give them a try!

The Bow. Using an oblong scarf, circle around your neck, making half a knot in the front. Keep one side longer than the other. Now, using the shorter end, form a loop. Wrap the longer end over the top of the loop and up behind it. Push the piece you are holding through the hole you just created. Pull both sides of the bow until they are even.

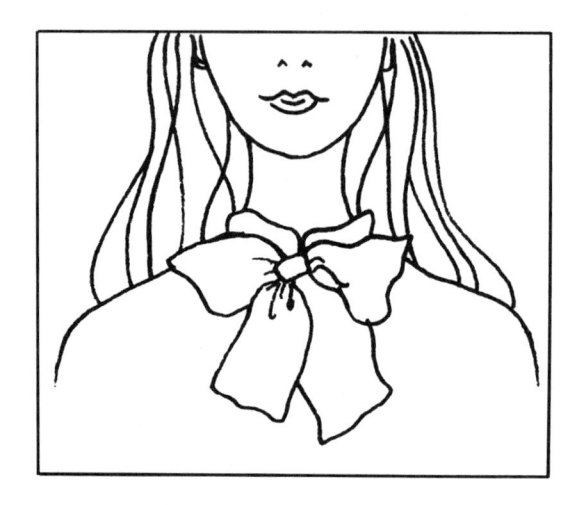

The Front Knot. Fold your square scarf in half, making a triangle. Bring the two longest ends around your neck to the front. Tie a knot. Fluff the ends. This can be tied at the base of your neck or lower. Try turning the scarf completely around, with the tip of the triangle in front.

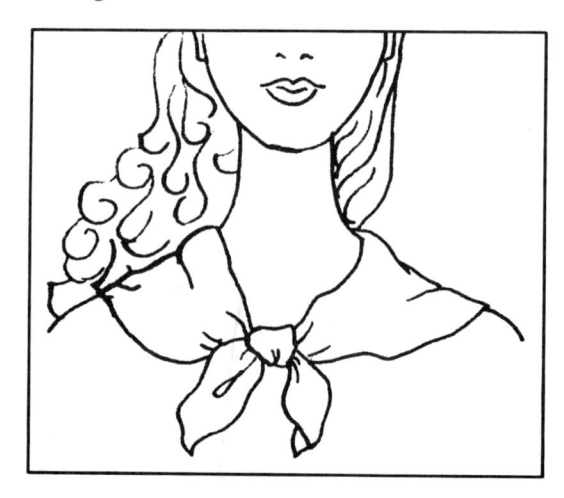

The Choker-Style Front Knot. This one is especially fun using a bandanna. Lay the scarf flat and fold the two opposite corners toward the center, creating one long piece. Tie a loose knot in the center. Place that knot at the front of your neck, tying it in the back. Adjust the length. Wear as shown or inside the open collar of a blouse.

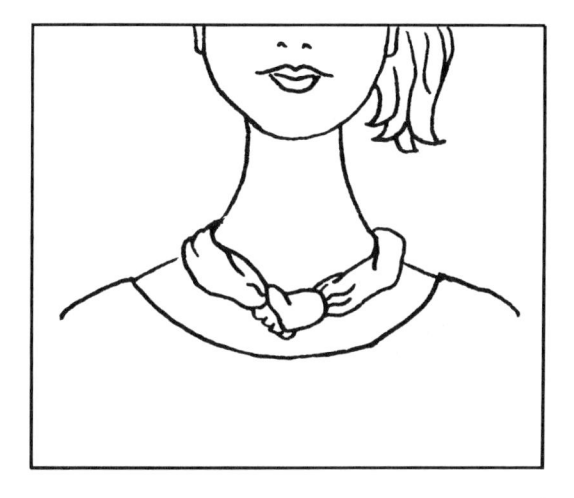

The Ascot. Using a square scarf, lay it out flat, wrong side up. Now make a knot in the center. Turn it inside out so the knot is inside. Take the opposite corners and tie around the back of your neck. Wear out or tucked inside your neckline.

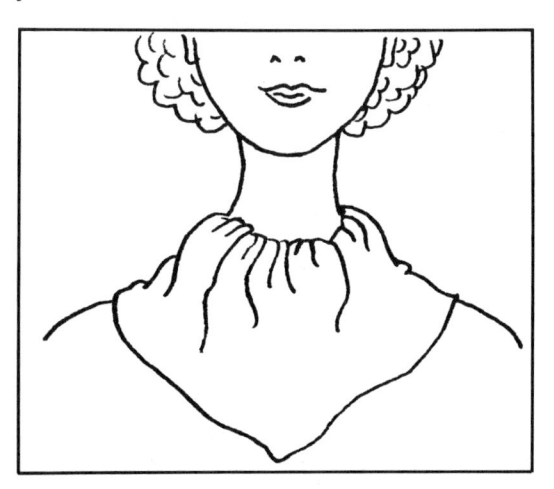

The Side Knot—Cowgirl Style. Fold a large square scarf into a triangle. Tie the opposite corners into a big loose knot over one shoulder. Fluff the ends. Away you go!

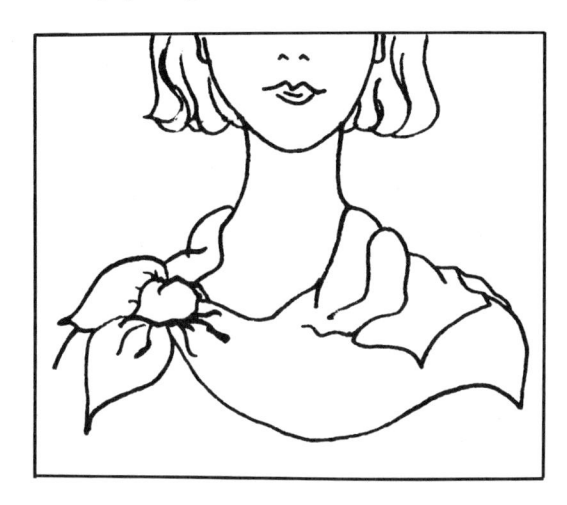

The Modified Man's Tie. Wrap an oblong scarf around your neck, leaving one side longer than the other. Use the longer side to wrap around the shorter side twice. Now bring it up through the V and tuck it down into the loop you created when you wrapped it up around the shorter side. Adjust the knot to the position you want.

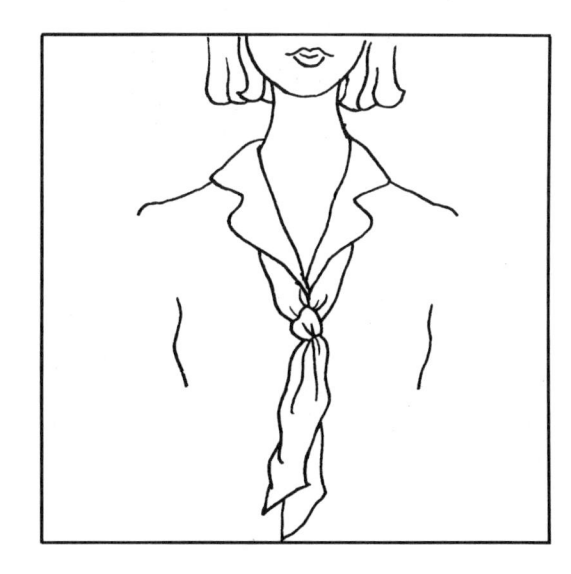

The Square-Knot Sash. Wrap your scarf around your waist, tying a square knot on the side. Let ends hang, tuck them under, or make a bow.

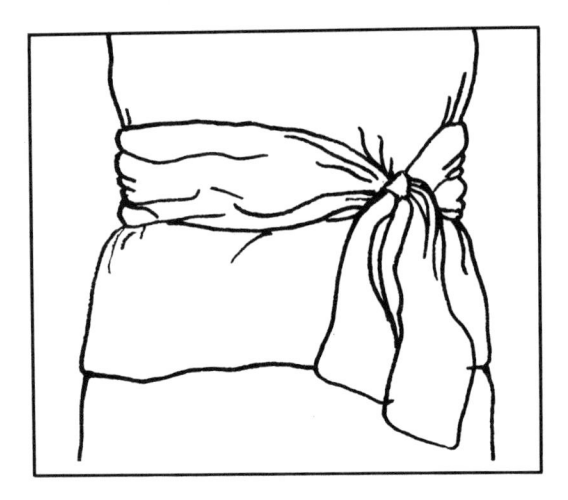

The Wrap-and-Tuck Sash. Depending on the length of your oblong scarf, single or double wrap the scarf around your waist. Twist the ends around each other in the front, tucking them under.

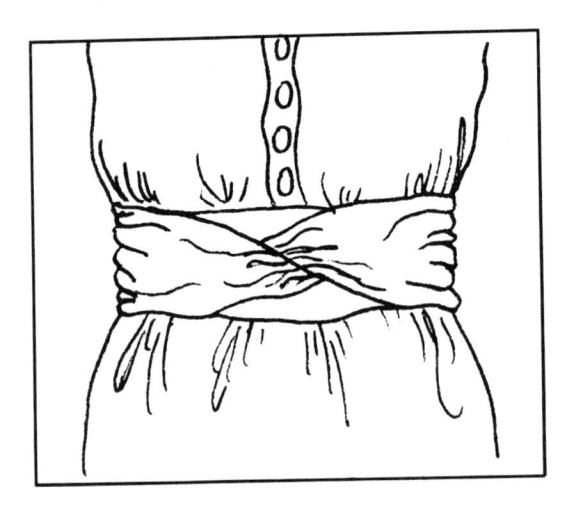

The Belt-Loop Belt. Use a rolled-up small square scarf as a belt. Pull it through your belt loops, tying it in the front. Bandannas are great for this, especially on your favorite jeans.

There are many more ways to tie scarves. Experiment and see what you can come up with!

Proper Care for Long-Lasting Wear

Caring for your clothes and accessories will help them last longer. Following are some handy suggestions. If you come across ideas not mentioned here, jot them down with this list so you can have a complete proper-care program.

For the benefit of the many students I have had who do not know how to do their own laundry, I have included washing, drying, and ironing instructions. You cannot depend on Mom to do your laundry forever! Plus, I'll let you in on a little secret. Parents are more willing to purchase clothes when they know you buy wisely and take good care of the garments you already have.

General Care

1. After wearing a garment, check for perspiration odor or stain. Then choose whether to wash it or rehang it. If in doubt, wash it!
2. Use proper hangers. Jackets, coats, better dresses, even blouses are best on padded or wide plastic hangers. They won't leave the marks that wire hangers do. Hang skirts and pants on the double-clamped or double-bar style. Attach at the waist. Folding pants and sweaters over wire hangers leaves an unwanted crease. (See Figure 10-11.)
3. Store sweaters neatly folded or rolled. Hanging sweaters can cause them to stretch out.
4. Use a sharp tool such as a knife, scissors, or razor blade to remove pills or tiny balls from sweaters.

FUNCTIONING FASHION

5. If your garments snag, use a knit picker to pull the thread or yarn through to the back side of the garment. Don't cut off the snag!
6. Keep your closet well ventilated for the sake of your clothes and shoes. Putting a room freshener in your closet is a good idea.
7. To remove lint, use a lint brush or masking tape.
8. Watch for loose buttons, splitting seams, hanging hems, or broken zippers. Repair and replace as soon as necessary.
9. Keep wet deodorants and perfumes away from garments. They may stain.
10. Pull a scarf over your head to protect your clothes from makeup stains when you dress. This is a well-known model's must!

Launder With Love—
Wash and Dry

11. To restore shape to a stretched-out garment, hand wash it, then let it dry flat on a towel. If the garment will not shrink, toss it in the dryer when it is almost completely dry—five minutes at most.
12. Use bleach on white clothes only. Wash separately in hot water. Rinse in warm water.
13. Separate light colors from dark. Wash lights in warm water, then follow with a cool rinse.
14. Wash dark colors in cold water to prevent fading. Dark colors get a cold rinse.
15. Follow directions on package of detergent so you use the right amount.
16. Hand wash delicate items such as nylons, undergarments, and sweaters in Woolite or a mild soap.
17. In most washing machines, fabric softeners are conveniently added before the wash cycle begins. If your machine isn't like this, pay

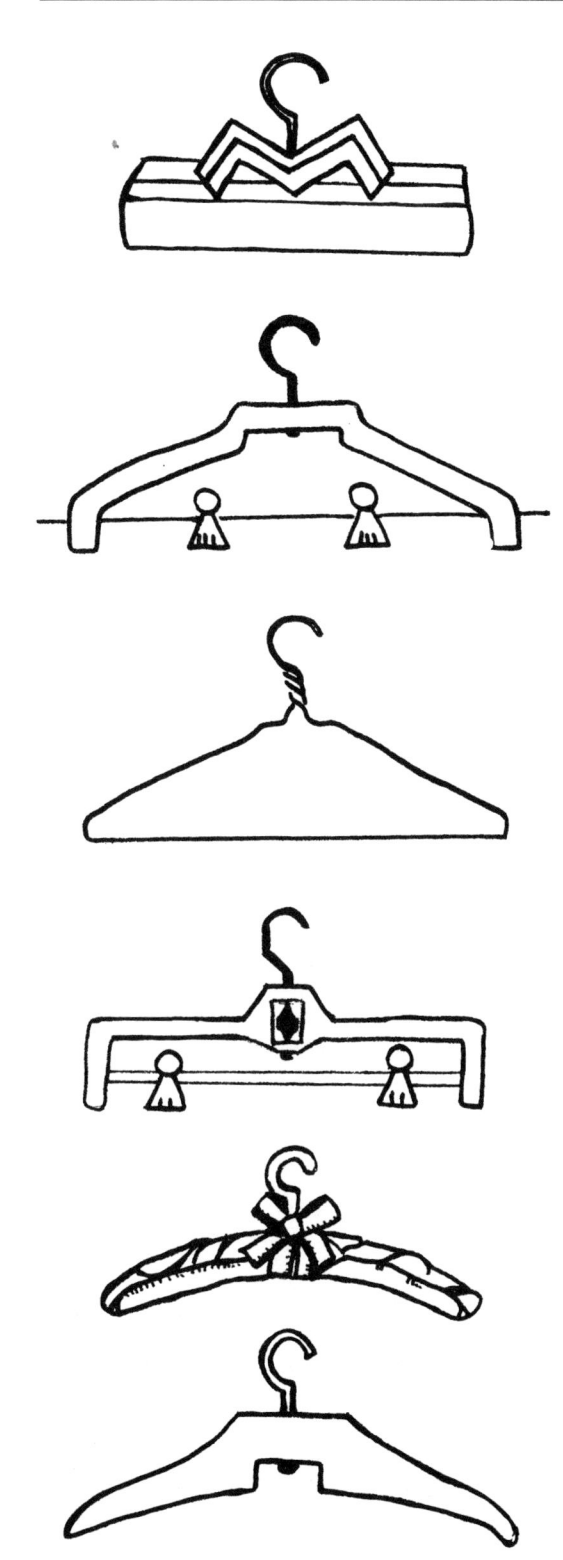

Figure 10-11. Use the proper hanger for effective results.

close attention to the cycle so you can add the softener at the appropriate time.
18. Carefully follow the instructions on clothing labels. Dry-clean when necessary or to prevent fading colors and worn-looking surfaces on certain fabrics.
19. Avoid dry-cleaning or washing one piece of a two-piece outfit without the other. Washing and dry-cleaning leaves garments looking different. You don't want to end up with your top faded from overwashing and your pants fresh and crisp from dry-cleaning.
20. If you air-dry clothes in the sun, turn them inside out to help prevent fading.

Stubborn Stains
21. Stains don't have to put an end to your clothes. Work them out! Test cleaning solution on a hidden seam or inner hem before trying it on the spot. You want to be sure the solution won't damage the fabric of your garment.
22. Put a white cotton cloth under the stained fabric to help absorb excess cleaning fluid. Dampen a clean white soft cloth with the cleaning fluid; press and lift rather than rubbing in on the spot.
23. Never iron over a stain. This may permanently set it into the fabric. Remove stains immediately. You'll have a better chance of getting them out.
24. Make use of prewash cleaning solutions and stain removers. Spray 'n Wash and Shout are well-known brands. Heavy stains may need a stronger product.

Pressing Your Pretties
25. Hang up your clothes immediately after undressing to save you from ironing out wrinkles later on. It means less wear and tear on fabrics, too.
26. Promptly remove clothes from the dryer and cut down on the amount of ironing you need to do.
27. Set the iron according to the type of fabric you are ironing. Most irons have a temperature guide right on them.
28. Iron lower-setting fabrics first so you don't have to stop and wait for the iron to cool.
29. Use Teflon-coated iron shields to make the job a bit smoother.
30. Spray starch gives fabric a new crispness and prolongs the start of wrinkles. Don't use starch on wools, corduroy, silks, or similar fabrics.
31. Try ironing corduroy, rayon, wool, velour, and other nap fabrics inside out for better-looking results.
32. Avoid smashing your clothes together in your closet. This will keep you from having to re-iron them before you wear them.
33. Iron around plastic buttons and metal zippers. Plastic buttons can melt and metal zippers get burning hot!
34. Iron small areas of a garment first: cuffs; collars, sleeves, waistbands, and pockets. Then go on to the larger areas. Always iron in the direction of the fabric's grain, not across it.
35. Hand-held steamers are perfect for traveling or quick touch-ups. Sure beats getting out the ironing board.

Dressed Outside— Dressed Inside

Make it a priority to dress for the Lord. You are in God's family, a royal family. Your clothing style and moderation can be used to reflect your love and consideration of God.

First Peter 3:3, 4 says our adornment or dressing should not be just outer but inner as well. We are to clothe our inner selves with the character of Christ.

First Peter 5:5 tells us to clothe ourselves with humility toward one another. We can choose to put on this attitude of humbleness. To be humble is to have a grateful appreciation of who God has created you to be: a servant, not to be served—having all of your actions and attitudes motivated by love.

Colossians 3:12–14 gives more guidelines for dressing your inner person. Put on a heart of compassion, it instructs. Compassion is having feelings of concern and love toward others, being able to see them and their struggles through eyes of understanding and love, and then being moved to take action to help them.

Just as we dress ourselves for daily activities, so we can dress for spiritual activities. The armor of God given to us in Ephesians 6:10–18 is our spiritual outfit. Dress in it every single day! You will be ready for any occasion.

Putting It All Together

The final look in the mirror should show you two things:

First, a well put-together outfit; clothes that are well coordinated and complementary to your face and figure. Check to be sure your bra straps, underwear lines, hem, and slip are neatly hidden away. Any wrinkles? Hopefully not! Are your accessories being worn with a sense of harmony in relation to the rest of your outfit? Are you wearing the right thing? Does your outfit fit the occasion you are about to attend? Your mirror will let you know!

Second, the reflection in the mirror should be a young lady who is confident of who she is because of Jesus' love for her. Does that mirror reflect a heart of compassion and humility? What about the character of Christ? Does the expression on your face tell of your special love relationship with the Lord?

You can wear lots of things, but wearing a warm smile far outweighs the latest fashion you might have on. A smile tells others of the joy in your heart. Let the joy that Jesus gives be shared. Put on a smile and wear it all day!

FUNCTIONING FASHION

Project Page

1. How can you create a wardrobe that functions more efficiently?

2. Go through the "Organizing Your Wardrobe" section step by step. What can you eliminate? What can you give away to someone who needs it more?

3. Take a look at your present wardrobe. What does it tell others about you? How does it reveal who you are? How does it not reveal who you are?

4. Answer each "Smart Shopper" question on page 159. You may find out you have some shopping habits to improve on! Try quality in your main garments and quantity in your less-expensive accessories.

5. Using the information given in this chapter, identify which of the following best fits you:

Figure
_____ hourglass
_____ inverted triangle
_____ triangle
_____ round
_____ square

_____ petite
_____ tall
_____ short-waisted
_____ long-waisted
_____ short neck
_____ long neck

Line
_____ horizontal
_____ vertical
_____ diagonal
_____ curved

Face
_____ oval
_____ round
_____ oblong
_____ square
_____ pear
_____ heart
_____ diamond
_____ rectangle

FUNCTIONING FASHION

6. Using this information, describe the styles of clothing and fabrics that will enhance your figure and face._____
_____
_____

7. Get your wardrobe in tip-top shape! Turn to page 162 and follow the closet organization plan laid out for you. Weed out, separate, and group your clothes. You may want to try adding a shelf, a shoe rack, or an extra rod to make your closet more functional.

8. Piece your wardrobe puzzle together! Fill in the chart on page 165. List the garments and the colors you need in order to make your wardrobe complete. Do the same with your accessories.

9. Change an outfit from daytime into dressy! Select a basic outfit. Change the accessories to give it a sporty daytime look, then a dressier look.

10. What would be an appropriate outfit for each of the following occasions:
    school_____
    church_____
    formal dance_____
    school sports event_____
    a casual date_____

11. Name three of your favorite labels or designers, and explain why they are your favorites._____
_____
_____
_____
_____

12. First Peter 3:4 instructs us to clothe ourselves inwardly. List three ways you can clothe your inner self with the character of Christ._____
_____
_____
_____

13. Read Ephesians 6:10–18 to see what your spiritual wardrobe is. In your own words, describe how you can wear each of these garments._____
_____
_____
_____
_____
_____

11 DELICATE DETAILS
The Secrets of Personal Grooming

There are several specifics of daily personal grooming that can't be overlooked. Here is a chance for you to show yourself how much you like you, by taking good care of yourself right down to the last intimate detail!

Undergarments

Always wear clean underclothes. Daily changing guarantees you the most sanitary approach to body discharges and odors. Be especially aware of changing your bra if you have exercised in it. And need I say, do wear a bra. Being seen without one can give others a negative impression.

Matching colored panties, bras, slips, and camisoles give a nice consistency and a prettier look to your underdressing. I feel more feminine in undergarments in flesh tones that have a satiny feel. Orange polka-dotted undies with a lavender bra just don't do it for me!

One half-slip, a whole slip, and a camisole are usually sufficient for your underclothes needs. Keep them freshly laundered. Wear a camisole under near-sheer blouses or scratchy wools.

Check to make sure your bra straps are not showing, panty lines aren't evident, and your slip is not peeking out from under your dress!

Mouth Matters

What a warm message you send when you smile! And what a good confident smile you can flash when you have sparkling teeth and fresh breath! Using a medium-soft toothbrush, brush several times a day! Brush the outside and the inside of your teeth. Turn your bristles at a forty-five-degree angle. Front inner teeth can then be brushed up and down, using your toothbrush vertically.

Your toothpaste needs to do more than just taste good! Use a brand with fluoride. Fluoride actively fights cavities.

Floss between teeth daily with unwaxed dental floss. Flossing can remove most bacterial plaque that builds up on teeth.

Brushing with baking soda helps remove stains from the enamel of your teeth.

Regular visits to the dentist is the best form of preventative care and can save you from gum disease and tooth decay in the future!

Use an effective mouthwash when needed. Nothing is more embarrassing than bad breath! It is a good idea to carry a breath-freshener spray in your purse or schoolbag.

A Bath a Day Keeps the Odor Away

A daily bath or shower will keep you clean and fresh-feeling throughout the day! A luxurious, steaming hot bath is wonderful for relaxing your muscles after a long day. Conditioning bubble baths are great fun and very moisturizing for your skin. Bath oils soften your skin and leave it feeling silky. Try a soothing herb tea bath for a delightful change—mint, sage, rosemary, or lemon. Keep the herbs from going down the drain by putting the loose tea in a tea bag or clean, loose-knit sock.

If you're in the mood for a real treat, how about a milk bath? Pour approximately one cup of milk powder flakes or one pint of milk into a full warm-watered tub. Enjoy!

Showering is much more practical on those get-up-late mornings before school. Cool showers in the A.M. will wake you up; a warmer temperature in the P.M. will relax you before bedtime. Daily showers are a must during your menstruation time. This is not the time for baths. Always give special attention to odorous areas.

Put an End to Rough Skin

While you are in the shower, use a pumice stone or foot scrub to remove tough, dead skin cells from your heels, inner ankles, and elbows. A loofah sponge mitt will take care of the unwanted cells on the rest of your body, as will an exfoliation product such as Clinique Body Scrub. Don't rub too hard. Your skin is delicate!

Bath Time Extras

Keep an old toothbrush or nailbrush handy for scrubbing your toenails. They get dirty! And you might as well do your fingernails while you're at it.

Hand-held massagers with rubber tips have become popular over the last several years. They originated in Europe, where massage is more common. Massagers are effective for muscle relaxation and cellulite stimulation. Many come with special creams to use after the massage. Follow the instructions given with your massager.

After-Bath Pampering— It Does a Body Good

While your skin is still warm and a bit damp, moisturize from neck to toe. Use a good nonperfumed body lotion. The lotion will seal in your natural moisture. Your shins, forearms, and shoulders will be very appreciative of this special care!

Those shoulders of yours also love being pampered with powder! Apply generously to shoulders, chest, and naturally odorous areas. Unscented powder is best if you plan on using cologne or perfume, unless you are using a dusting powder from your fragrance line. You don't want your scents to clash!

Underarm Protection

Deodorants and antiperspirants are not the same. Deodorants decrease odor, antiperspirants decrease wetness. Some products include both. Use these products in conjunction with your needs.

Not all people need both. It depends upon your individual body chemistry, rate of perspiration, and amount of odor. Sweating and smelling are natural. No need to feel dirty or embarrassed. If you are unable to reapply deodorant or antiperspirant after working out, at least dab on extra cologne for the time being. Deodorants are usually needed when puberty attacks! Your body changes drastically, and this is one of the results. Roll-on wet, roll-on dry, spray, stick, or cream; take your pick, there are many forms available! If your deodorant or antiperspirant should cause a rash, stop using it and choose another.

Removing Unwanted Hair

Make my shave a close one! Shaving is the most common form of hair removal from legs and underarms. I love the feel of freshly shaved legs! Use a double-edged razor and soapsuds or shaving cream. Pressing too hard may cause you to slice your skin. Ouch!

Repeating this twice a week is usually sufficient, but it will depend on your rate of hair growth. The nubs that grow back feel prickly because the razor blunt-cuts the hair. Not so with waxing.

Wax Away!

Waxing is a form of hair removal that has longer-lasting results. It is more expensive and time-consuming during the actual process, and semi-painful. Waxing pulls the hairs out, roots and all, so it takes four to six weeks for the fine new hairs to reappear above the surface. Salon waxing is safer and easier, though many girls wax at home.

Facial waxing is the best way to remove unwanted hair on your face. Stray hairs between eyebrows, upper lip, and even chin and cheek sideburn areas require waxing for some. Be sure the appropriate procedure is done. I have had skin ripped off my face from incorrect waxing. Never shave facial hair! Hot-wax and cold-wax methods are now available. The preference is yours.

Cream Away!

Cream depilatories are another form of hair removal. The hair is actually dissolved by the cream. Needless to say, this can be irritating to the skin. I have never used these products because I can imagine the harshness of the chemicals used.

Shock Away!

Electrolysis is the only permanent form of hair removal. A fine needle is inserted into the hair follicle, and then a low voltage of electricity is applied. The electricity destroys the follicle and papilla (new hair). This process is expensive and painful.

Bleach Away!

Bleaching is a way of lightening facial hair if you choose not to remove it. Follow the directions carefully, making sure your skin is not blemished where you want to bleach.

Heavenly Scent

The fragrance you choose to wear is a very personal matter. What appeals to you is often an expression of your personal statement. Fragrances range from fresh florals, fruits, and spices to meadowy, woodsy, and exotic scents, including even designer originals. Some are heavy; some are light.

I believe a woman should select her fragrance based on her own preference. Many advertisements suggest selecting a scent that will please the man in your life. Well, maybe, but I'm the one who enjoys my fragrance and smells it much more than my husband does. As a single woman, I certainly didn't rely on my fragrance to attract dates!

Test new fragrances one at a time before you buy them. Either ask for a sample or dab the fragrance on your forearm and then walk around the store so the cologne can adjust itself to your body chemistry. Your unique body oils will determine the smell of the fragrance. You may like it more or less after wearing it for an hour or so. This also allows time to see if you react negatively to the scent. Having demonstrated fragrances in a department store for many years, I know the reaction of a fragrance that does not agree with me: headache, nausea, and stuffy nose!

The lasting ability of your fragrance again depends on your personal body oils and heat, and also on the form of the fragrance you use. Perfume is oil based and concentrated, so its staying power is much longer than cologne or toilet water. Cologne is alcohol based, evaporates quickly, and is less concentrated. Toilet water is water based and is the least concentrated. It is lightly scented and can be used generously. Toilet waters are often referred to as "splash."

Put It Where It Counts

The best places to apply your fragrance are the warm spots of your body: behind your ears, near the nape of your neck, on your inner elbows, your wrists, on your stomach, and on your temples. However, remember that applying fragrance on your wrists is useless if you find yourself washing your hands all day. You are bound to rinse off the scent. Your body heat gives the fragrance its full blossoming potential. Since heat rises, placing fragrance on your stomach is good strategy. Just don't overdo it. Others shouldn't be able to smell you coming down the hall!

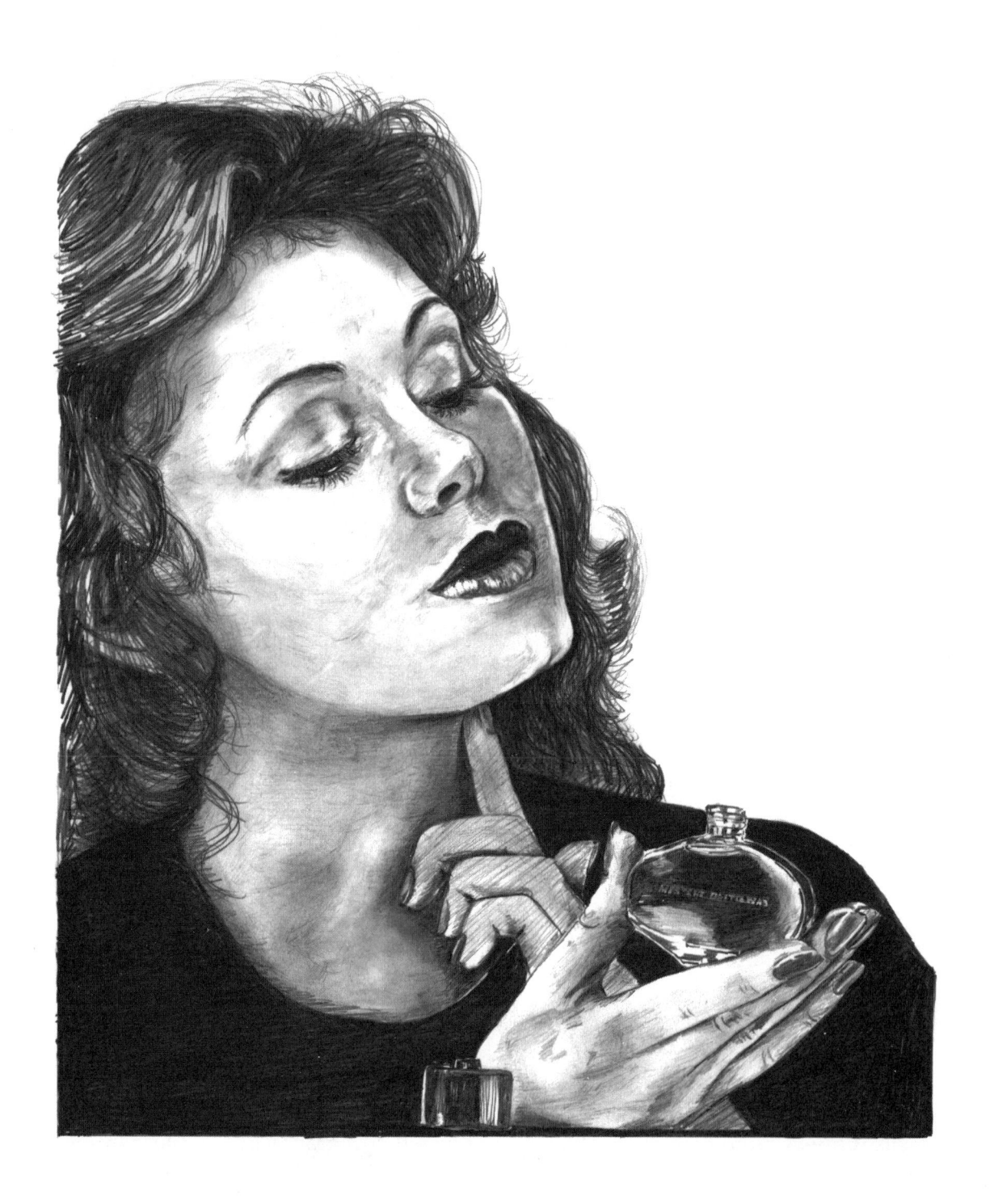

BEAUTIFULLY CREATED

Long-Lasting Layering

Fragrance layering is another way of keeping your fragrance throughout the day. Scented bath gel, body lotion, and dusting powder followed by a spray of cologne or a touch of perfume work beautifully. They must, however, be the same scent! This approach is not necessary and can be tough on the budget. It does give you a sense of femininity, though. Carry an atomizer or purse spray with you for instant touch-ups during the day.

Surrounded by Scents!

Surround yourself with pretty scents by using room fresheners. Small perfumed soaps are great for tantalizing lingerie drawers, closets, bathrooms, or suitcases. Try misting a few cotton balls with fragrance, let dry, then tuck them in your traveling bags, purse, or pillowcase!

A Sweet Aroma

Fragrances enhance, uplift, and make more enjoyable the presence of the person wearing them. Did you know that you are a fragrance? That's right. The Bible says that as Christians we are a sweet aroma, a fragrance of Christ to God. The sweet scent we release is to be evident among those who are unbelievers, according to 2 Corinthians 2:15. Our aroma is proof that Christ is in us. Our fragrance enhances, encourages, and delights others. Our sweet scent is a constant glory to our Lord.

DELICATE DETAILS
Project Page

1. Analyze your undergarments. Are you in need of new underwear—a slip, perhaps a bra or camisole?

2. See if you can pass the "Mouth Matters" test. Check which of the following you do regularly:
   _____ brush your teeth
   _____ use a fluoride toothpaste
   _____ floss
   _____ use mouthwash
   _____ carry a purse-size breath freshener
   _____ visit your dentist regularly

   Scores: 6 out of 6 = excellent; 5 out of 6 = good; 4 out of 6 = fair; 3 or below = may need improvement!

3. Complete this sentence. A steaming hot bath is best at_____ to relax, and a_____ shower is best in the morning to wake yourself up!

4. Deodorants stop odor, antiperspirants stop wetness. Which do you need? Which form do you prefer—stick, roll-on wet, roll-on dry, spray, or cream?_____
   _____
   _____
   _____

5. Match the form of fragrance with its base ingredient.
   _____ perfume   _____ water
   _____ cologne   _____ oil
   _____ toilet   _____ alcohol

6. Circle the fragrance type you think best fits your personality:
   fruity, floral, spicy, woodsy, meadowy.

7. According to 2 Corinthians 2:15, we are to God as a fragrance of Christ. What scent are you releasing to others?

12 INNER BEAUTY
Beauty Through and Through

In my younger days, I was totally obsessed with beauty. I stared at magazine covers and gorgeous makeup and hair advertisements all the time. Beautiful-looking people really had it all together. They had an upper hand on life. At least that's what I thought.

It was when I was modeling in New York that God opened my eyes to see the true definition of the word *beauty*. Actually, the whole lesson centered around Janice. Here's what happened.

The test board at Wilhelmina consisted of the new models. We were the ones who were green to the business. We spent most of our time taking test pictures, hoping to put together a dynamic portfolio. That's where I met Janice. She had been with the agency a little longer than I had. Janice was one of those girls with thick, bouncy hair, straight white teeth, flawless skin, tiny hips, and an upper body that just couldn't be missed. You know. She was one of those girls everyone else wished they looked like.

Well, one afternoon after I had been test shooting, I stopped in at the agency. The room buzzed with ringing telephones, busy bookers, and a few models, one of whom was Janice. The attention, as usual, centered on her. Everyone seemed to be in awe of Janice's sudden weight loss. I listened to her exaggerated explanation of how "it was nothing." She had just taken up jogging and quit eating so much. "After all," she exclaimed, "what is there worth eating anyway?"

Are you kidding? If New York doesn't make you fat, nothing will. Every corner has a vendor selling some sort of tempting tasty. Trail mix, roasted cashews, hot dogs, and—can you believe it—pizza by the slice! I was pudging out underneath my oversized sweater, but not Janice. No way. She had taken up jogging. I had tried jogging, too. I jogged two blocks up to the Bagel Nosh, got two cinnamon-raisin bagels to go, and jogged back. Obviously, Janice and I were not using the same method of jogging!

As I sat there listening, the subject changed to Janice's new boyfriend and how hot his body was. Janice's language became crude and I began to feel uncomfortable. The longer I looked and listened, the more unattractive she became. Her beauty began to crumble before my eyes.

Off to her next appointment, Janice strutted out of the room. That's when the truth about her weight loss was uncovered. "Want to know what I heard about Janice's 'Oh, it was nothing' weight loss?" one of the models asked in a daring tone of voice. "Janice didn't sweat one drop to lose a pound. She just popped pills." She paused. "Speed." A hush came over the room. Drugs? And to think I had thought she had it all. Janice looked great on the outside, but inside there was nothing.

I learned a lesson that day: Outer beauty is a waste if there is no inner beauty to go with it. It's like having an elegant hand-cut crystal vase with no flowers in it—empty. True beauty is more than being able to offer the world a frosty smile on the cover of a magazine. It means being a person who is honest and cares for others—a person who can laugh and cry with others. That is true beauty. That's what I want.

What Is Inner Beauty?

When I ask girls what their definition of *inner beauty* is, many tell me they think of someone who is kind, unselfish, and loving toward others. Maybe, you would say, a person with inner beauty is one who is always happy, goes to church, and is nice to kids at school—even to the ones no one else likes.

Well, all of these are correct. They each describe loving and thoughtful actions rather than appearance. Inner beauty is not based on what you look like but what you act like.

Think about the important people in your life. Are they special because of what they look like? No, it's probably because of their kindness, loyalty, friendship, or maybe because they are always there when you need them. It's because of their inner beauty.

Jesus was like that. People didn't like Him because He was tall, dark, and handsome. It was because of the person He was on the inside. Isaiah 53:2 tells us, "He [Jesus] has no form or comeliness that we should look at Him, and no beauty that we should desire Him" (AMP).

You mean that Jesus wasn't the suave, macho-type like the guys you daydream about? No. What was it, then, that caused people to be drawn to Him by the thousands? What made Jesus so magnetic? His inner beauty.

Jesus was kind to the poor woman at the well. He traveled miles to lay hands on people who were sick. He came along at the right moment to assist fishermen with their catch for the day.

He made time in His busy schedule to eat a meal with those who needed His forgiveness. He served others by providing food for all those people and by washing the disciples' feet. He gave of Himself to show that He cared. Ultimately He gave everything: He gave His life for us.

It wasn't Jesus' appearance that made Him beautiful. It was His heart.

What's in a person's heart will affect the amount of inner beauty he or she has. Usually what is in our hearts determines what our actions will be. Do you have a heart filled with love or hatefulness, forgiveness or resentment, caring or indifference, joyfulness or depression?

The Lord is keeping watch over our hearts. First Samuel 16:7 says, "God sees not as man sees, for man looks at the outward appearance, but the Lord looks at the heart." It's true that we notice the outer appearance of others first. Then we get to know them and we can see their inner appearance, their hearts. That's where God looks first. He really wants us to be beautiful on the inside. He wants us to act in loving ways—to be a reflection of His love and His image. He wants our hearts to be filled with consideration, contentment, and consistency. These are three key building blocks to inner beauty.

Building Blocks to Inner Beauty

Consideration

Katie had worked earnestly in anticipation of this day. Fancy footsteps, routines, high kicks, enthusiastic smiles—she had mastered them all in hopes of winning the judges' favor. Cheerleading tryouts were today.

When Katie arrived early at the old gym, where the tryouts were to be held, she drew a number from the big fish bowl to see where she would fall in tryout order. Number two. She was thrilled. This would give her a chance to perform for the judges before almost all of the other girls. It meant everything to Katie to make it as a cheerleader, and being number two was more than she could have asked for.

The other girls arrived. Some were excited, some scared. But all were frantically practicing cheers under their breath.

Katie looked at her watch. Only a few more minutes, and her big moment would be here.

Anxiously looking around, Katie noticed Peggy, a friend from English class, standing away from the others. Peggy looked rather distressed. Surely something wasn't right. Katie was bothered by Peggy's appearance. She made her way through swinging arms and kicking legs over to Peggy.

"Hi Peggy," Katie greeted her. "Oh, hi Katie," Peggy responded quickly, without looking up.

"Gee, Peggy, everyone is so excited about tryouts. They're practicing like crazy. Did you want to practice? I mean, if you need help with a cheer, I could help you real quick." Katie rushed the words out, knowing tryouts were about to start.

"No thanks, Katie. I know the cheers pretty well. That's not the problem." Peggy lifted her eyes to look at Katie. "I just found out that my grandpa was rushed to the hospital and I want to get over there, but I've worked so hard for the tryouts. I've always wanted to be a cheerleader. And can you believe, I'm number twenty-seven out of twenty-nine girls trying out." Peggy's glanced dropped. "I don't know if I can wait that long."

Katie instantly felt a pang in her stomach. She cared about Peggy and knew how awful she must feel. But if she traded her number she might ruin her chances at making the cheerleading squad. *Well,* she thought, *if I make it, I make it. If I don't, I don't.* Peggy's grandfather was more important than wanting to perform first.

"Listen Peggy, I drew number two. Why don't we trade numbers—then you can get over to the hospital and be with your grandpa."

"Really?" Peggy asked in a hopeful voice.

"Yeah, really," Katie smiled.

"Number two," the squad director shouted from the other end of the gym. Katie handed her number to Peggy. After a quick hug, Peggy darted toward the tryout room. Just to see her so excited was worth the trade-off to Katie.

Katie was considerate of Peggy's feelings. She was aware of her needs. Being aware of others' feelings and needs are true inner-beauty qualities. Some people are too wrapped up in their own lives to even notice that someone else is hurting or in need.

Considerate people notice, but they do more than that. They do something about it! They go ahead and help when it's needed, hug when it comforts, and often do the odd little jobs no one else wants to do.

Considerate people are not selfish. They are willing to put others before themselves. They are kind, loving, and willing to get involved in others' lives. Being considerate of others is a quality that enhances relationships and develops inner beauty.

Contentment

Contentment is a characteristic that is found in inwardly attractive people. Being content means being pleased and thankful for who you are and what you have. Content people can gracefully accept life's ups and downs, always seeming to make the best out of every situation.

When you are content on the inside, you have a true sense of joy and peace deep within you. Smiles come easily. Encouraging others seems natural. Loving life is your way of life.

Being happy with yourself and your life lets you focus your attention on others rather than worrying about yourself.

Do you know people who are content? Aren't they peaceful and calming to be around? They really help us keep our focus on the things that matter, especially the Lord. People with inner beauty are people others want to spend their time with. And one of the reasons is that they have learned to be content.

Consistency

Consistency is one of those words with a heavy-duty meaning. Karen found that out the hard way. She used to always shop and go for ice cream with Jamie. Recently she had been saying no to Jamie when she just didn't feel like going. Rather than being honest and being a good friend, she just told Jamie "No, I don't want ice cream today."

Jamie felt confused. She and Karen had been friends for years. They could always count on each other. When they spent time together, they talked about everything. Because Karen had become wishy-washy, Jamie felt hurt. She wasn't sure anymore if Karen was such a good friend. When they were together, Jamie felt reluctant to share things with Karen. She had lost trust in her. It is difficult to confide in someone who is your friend one minute but not the next. Eventually Jamie stopped calling Karen and made new friends.

Karen had really lost out. She valued Jamie's friendship but wasn't committed enough to be there when Jamie called. Karen had not been consistent in her actions and friendship with Jamie.

Consistency may be the hardest to develop of the three inner-beauty qualities. Being wishy-washy, moody, noncommitted, and unpredictable are the opposites of being consistent. The "yo-yo" person who is up and down, yes and no, or maybe so, will have a harder time building trust and respect in friendships with others. People who are consistent are people you can count on. They are people who are confident in being themselves—no masks, no games.

Consistency takes practice. We don't always feel like acting the same or following through on what we say we will do. That's why being consistent is a decision you make, not a feeling.

Jesus is consistent. He isn't loving one minute, mean the next. He doesn't act like a friend to your face and then talk behind your back. He doesn't act concerned with your troubles and then not care. He is consistent. That is one reason we can trust Him.

Like consideration and contentment, consistency can be learned. We can decide to embrace all three of these inner-beauty qualities and follow through on them with our actions. However, this whole process is much easier with the help of the Holy Spirit. The Holy Spirit oversees the construction process going on inside of you and me, building a more beautiful person on the inside.

Under Construction

In my own development of inner beauty, I have often asked, "Why do I always feel I am under construction? Will I ever really be beautiful on the inside?" When I grow in one area, the Lord shines His spotlight on another, and the inner-beauty construction process begins all over again. It is a journey. We are continuously under construction. The Holy Spirit works with us to build beauty from the inside outward. People who are filled with beauty on the inside radiate beauty on the outside, no matter what they look like physically.

I encourage you never to give up during the construction process. There are times you will want to toss in the towel—but don't. Holly didn't. Hanging in there sure paid off for her.

Holly heard about Jesus at a Christian camp, and became a Christian soon after. The decision to follow Christ seemed easy enough at the time, but now she was finding it shaky to be sixteen and to live for Jesus. She felt so discouraged she just wanted to quit. "Why does it matter what I act like and what I do?" she wanted to know.

Holly's Bible-study group met for breakfast before school on Wednesday mornings. They were in the middle of a study on the fruits of the Spirit when Holly started questioning herself. Love, joy, peace, patience. That's the one that stumped her: patience. She was having a hard time learning to be patient. Where was patience when she needed it the most? She needed it at home with her mom.

For the past couple of weeks, Holly's mom had really been getting on her nerves. She couldn't figure out why her mom was always telling her what to do. "Load the dishwasher, unload the dryer, clean your bedroom, dust the living room, finish your homework, baby-sit for the Stewarts so we can go to dinner with them, help your little brother with the trash." She never got the answer she wanted when she asked her mother, "But why?" "Because I said so," was not the answer she was looking for from her mom.

One night after a major explosion with her mother, Holly ran crying into her room. She slammed the door behind her. "Help me, Lord, I need more patience," she pleaded as she threw herself down on her bed. Holly really needed that patience she was learning about. Every time she spouted off to her mom, it made her feel ugly inside.

Holly could feel the Holy Spirit working to remind her to be patient. Suddenly the thoughts that came to her seemed to be just what she needed.

Holly knew from her Bible study that God wanted her to be patient. So, she must work *with* the Lord rather than *against* Him. She needed to decide to act patient in the situations with her mom. It made sense to her. Holly thought back to the fight she just had with her mother. If only she had chosen to be patient, as the Holy Spirit was prompting her to do, instead of acting angry, as her feelings were telling her to do, the scene with her mom might have been totally different.

Holly's sense of discouragement began to lift. As the days went on she had plenty of opportunity to try out her theory. What a surprise! It worked.

Patience grew in Holly. She didn't feel so ugly on the inside. She felt better about herself and her new way of acting. Holly's patience on the inside was making her prettier on the outside. She could feel the construction under way, for with the Lord's help she could act patiently.

Two Scriptures are helping me through the inner-beauty construction process. Psalms 138:8 says, "The Lord will perfect that which concerns me" (AMP). Philippians 1:6 adds, "For I am confident of this very thing, that He who began a good work in you will perfect it until the day of Christ Jesus."

Isn't that good news? God is doing good work in you and is perfecting all the things concerning you. And it never stops! The construction continues as you and the Lord work on building your inner self.

Beholding His Beauty

God's Word is His love letter to us. Reading that letter provides you with an opportunity to spend some very special time with Jesus. The more you know about Him, the more time you will want to spend with Him through reading and prayer. The more time you spend with Jesus, the more you become like Him and the more His beauty fills you.

Psalms 27:4 makes this point clear: "One thing I have asked from the Lord, that I shall seek: That I may dwell in the house [presence] of the Lord all the days of my life, To behold the beauty of the Lord, And to meditate in His temple."

When you spend time in the Lord's presence and think about what it says in His Word, you, like Jesus, will shine with a beauty that comes from within. This kind of beauty is lasting beauty.

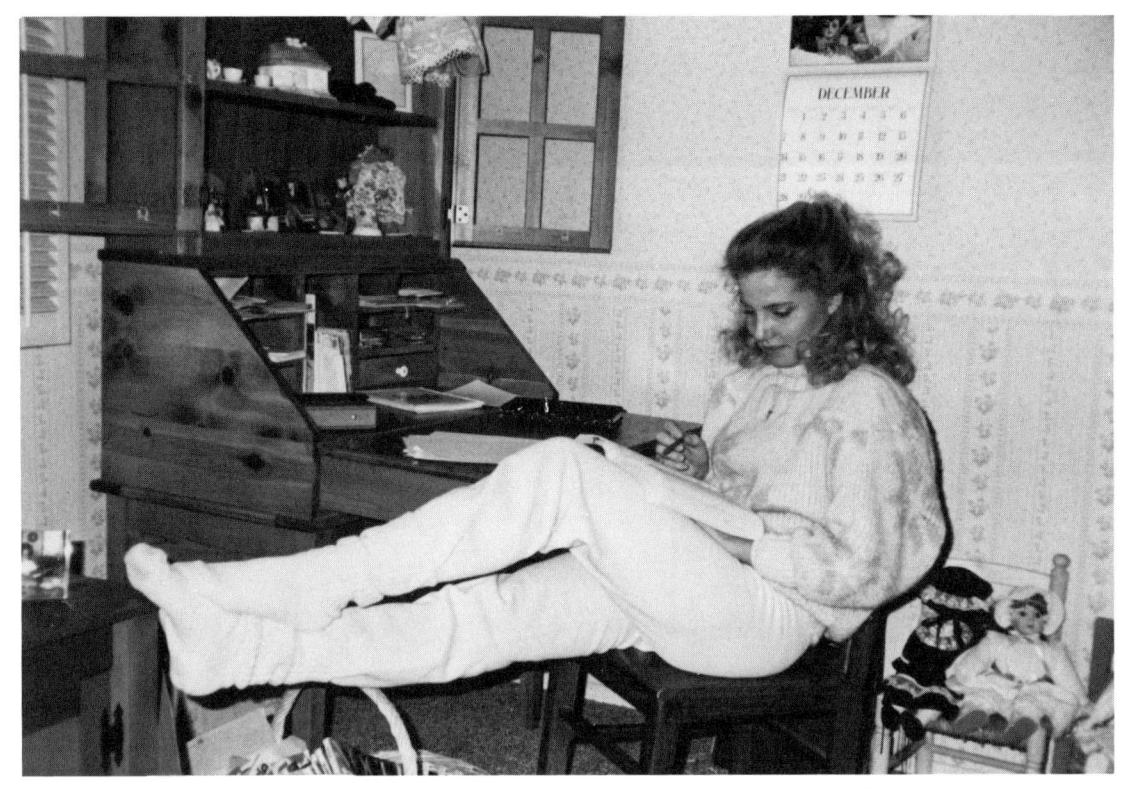

Make time each day to read God's Word, His personal love letter to you.

Second Corinthians 4:16 tells us that our outer appearance fades with age, but our inner self, our spirit, is made new and younger every day. Inner beauty that comes from spending time with Jesus will last forever.

No amount of makeup, skin care, classy colors, or clothes can give you the confidence and inner beauty that Jesus can. All of His qualities are available to you because His Spirit came to live inside you when you accepted Jesus into your heart. Developing inner beauty is possible for all of us if we allow the Holy Spirit to play an active part in our lives.

Beauty Takes Time

God has made us many promises worth hanging on to. One of them is this: God makes everything beautiful in His own time (Ecclesiastes 3:11 AMP). This includes you and me. You will get there, and the ending will make the journey worth its ups and downs.

You may be familiar with the words to the song "In His Time." It is by far one of my favorite songs. One day I was on my way to Bible study to play my guitar and lead the singing. A third verse to this song came to me. It goes like this:

In Your time,
In Your time,
You are making me beautiful
In Your time.
Lord, I pray to You this day
I'll reflect You in every way,
And I'll be just what you say
In Your time.

Make it your prayer. Hang the familiar phrase out on your construction site today.

Be patient. God's not finished with me yet!

And aren't you glad? Give Him time and give yourself time!

You are God's work of art. He has designed you on the outside and He is continually designing you on the inside, creating both inner and outer beauty. You *are* beautiful.

INNER BEAUTY

Project Page

1. In your own words, define *beauty*—both inner and outer.

2. Describe a person you know who has inner beauty. What does she act like, look like, and do for others?

3. Read Isaiah 53:2. Was Jesus physically attractive to people? What was it that attracted people to Him?

4. Now read Proverbs 4:23. The contents of our hearts will determine our actions. So, why is it important for us to "watch over our hearts"?

5. Are you aware of the feelings and needs of those closest to you? List the names of your family members. Next to their names jot down what you think their needs are. How can you help fulfill those needs?

6. Being content means being pleased and thankful for who you are and what you have. Contentment leads to peace and joy. Write a paragraph explaining why you are or are not content with your life. _____
_____
_____
_____
_____
_____

7. Define *consistency*. Write a brief description of a friend who is consistent and another who is inconsistent. Which one can you count on? Which are you? _____
_____
_____
_____
_____
_____

8. Like Holly, we are all under the inner beauty construction process. How is the Holy Spirit working to build inner beauty into your life? _____
_____
_____
_____

9. Spending time in God's presence, in prayer, and in reading the Bible will help you shine with a beauty that comes from within. Make a decision today to spend time with Jesus as often as you can—maybe even every day.

   Use the following chart as your personal Bible reading plan. When you complete a chapter in each book of the Bible, check it off. It will be fun to watch your progress.

THE NEW TESTAMENT

Matthew	1	2	3	4	5	6	7	8	9	10	11	12	13	14	15	16
	17	18	19	20	21	22	23	24	25	26	27	28				
Mark	1	2	3	4	5	6	7	8	9	10	11	12	13	14	15	16
Luke	1	2	3	4	5	6	7	8	9	10	11	12	13	14	15	16
	17	18	19	20	21	22	23	24								
John	1	2	3	4	5	6	7	8	9	10	11	12	13	14	15	16
	17	18	19	20	21											
Acts	1	2	3	4	5	6	7	8	9	10	11	12	13	14	15	16
	17	18	19	20	21	22	23	24	25	26	27	28				
Romans	1	2	3	4	5	6	7	8	9	10	11	12	13	14	15	16
1 Corinthians	1	2	3	4	5	6	7	8	9	10	11	12	13	14	15	16
2 Corinthians	1	2	3	4	5	6	7	8	9	10	11	12	13			
Galatians	1	2	3	4	5	6										
Ephesians	1	2	3	4	5	6										
Philippians	1	2	3	4												
Colossians	1	2	3	4												
1 Thess.	1	2	3	4	5											
2 Thess.	1	2	3													
1 Timothy	1	2	3	4	5	6										
2 Timothy	1	2	3	4												
Titus	1	2	3													
Philemon	1															
Hebrews	1	2	3	4	5	6	7	8	9	10	11	12	13			
James	1	2	3	4	5											
1 Peter	1	2	3	4	5											
2 Peter	1	2	3													
1 John	1	2	3	4	5											
2 John	1															
3 John	1															
Jude	1															
Revelation	1	2	3	4	5	6	7	8	9	10	11	12	13	14	15	16
	17	18	19	20	21	22										

SELF-IMAGE PROGRESS REPORT

Since the time you began reading this book, has your self-image improved? Fill in the following progress report to find out. For best results, be honest with yourself!

1. Which of the following low self-image symptoms does *not* describe you?
   _____ I have a pimple; I'd better hide.
   _____ If I were prettier, I'd have more dates.
   _____ Everybody is better than me.
   _____ Guess jeans make me fit in.
   _____ My appearance is all wrong.
   _____ God wasn't paying attention when He made me.
2. Of the following young women, who do you wish you were?
   _____ Molly Ringwald   _____ Princess Diana
   _____ Amy Grant   _____ Kim Fields
   _____ Miss Teen USA   _____ Myself
3. Check the physical features you would like to change.
   _____ nose   _____ body frame
   _____ eyes   _____ hair
   _____ face shape   _____ none
   _____ mouth   _____ teeth
   _____ freckles, moles   _____ hands, nails
4. Which is most important to you?
   _____ your wardrobe
   _____ your appearance
   _____ your popularity
   _____ being yourself
5. Answer yes or no to the next two questions.
   a. Do you believe God loves you just the way He designed you?
      _____ yes   _____ no
   b. Are you learning to like the way God made you?
      _____ yes   _____ no
6. Rank the following in order of importance.
   _____ what others say about me
   _____ how I feel about myself
   _____ what God's Word says about me
7. What plans have you made to become the inwardly beautiful person God wants you to be? Check one or more.
   _____ None.
   _____ I've started to read the Bible.
   _____ I am praying more often.
   _____ I am confessing my sins daily.
   _____ I am learning to be content, consistent, considerate, and confident.

8. Answer the following true or false.
    _____ God is on my side.
    _____ God has a special plan for my life.
    _____ If I were the only person alive, Jesus still would have died for me.
    _____ I am valuable.
    _____ I am beautiful in God's eyes.
    _____ Nobody is a nobody, especially me.

Well, how did you do? Go back and reread each question and your answer. Has your answer improved over the answer you would have given before reading this book? What percentage has it improved: 10 percent, 25 percent, 50 percent, 75 percent, or 100 percent? Pray and ask God to help you to keep working on improving your self-image. You are very important to Him and He is always there for you.

Perhaps you can share this report with an older Christian you trust. Ask him or her to pray with you.

Dear Friend,

One of the greatest times in my life was when I began to understand God's unconditional love for me. It honestly changed my life.

Realizing I was loved and forgiven enabled me to open my heart to the Lord's cleansing and healing power. I was able to view myself through new eyes. I can now see myself as having value—not because of what I've done or haven't done but just because Jesus loves me and accepts me. He created me, died for me, and offered me life forever with Him in heaven. He has done the same for you.

Have you received God's love, forgiveness, and eternal life? If not, please do it today. How? By asking Jesus into your heart to be your Savior, then by going one step further and making Him your Lord—allowing Him to lay out the plan for your life. Choosing to become part of the family of God and having a personal relationship with Jesus will be the most important decision of your life.

Will you pray this prayer with me?

> Dear Heavenly Father,
> I come to You right now with an open heart. I do believe that Jesus is Your Son, that He died for me and rose from the dead. Jesus, please send Your Spirit to live inside of me, to guide me and be my friend forever. I know I haven't always done the right things, but the Bible says You forgive me when I sincerely ask You to. So Lord, please forgive me, cleanse me, and heal the hurt deep inside. Lord, I give my life to You. Thank You for loving me and giving me a new beginning. I pray this in Jesus' name. Amen.

If you just prayed this prayer for the first time, congratulations! You just became a Christian. Will you write and tell me about it today? Jesus loves you and I do, too.

In Jesus,

Andrea

INDEX

Acne, 56. *See also* Skin breakout; Skin care
Aerobic exercise, 92–95
  tips on, 96
  nonaerobic exercise, 96, 97
Alcohol, 76, 84, 85
American Look, The, 16
Anorexia nervosa, 76
Astringent, 48, 50–53, 111

Balance, 35–37
Bandy, Way, 62, 63
Base, 63. *See also* Foundation
Bathing, 181, 182
Beauty, inner, 187, 188
  personified by Christ, 188, 189
  characteristics of, 189–191
  progressing toward, 191–194, 197
Blow drying, 127–129
Blush, 49, 62, 68–72, 111, 150
Body
  types, 29
  alignment, 34
  weight, 77
  shape, 97
  measurement chart, 110
  size and hairstyle, 120
  use of color, 151
  fashion styles, 161, 162
Brushing hair, 118, 119, 127, 130
Bulimia, 76
Bust line, 36, 151, 161

Christ, Jesus
  trusting in, 19–21, 33, 54, 76, 83–86, 113, 114, 141, 157, 191, 200
  getting to know, 37, 38, 61, 85, 86, 192–194, 197
  representing to others, 41, 63, 65, 71, 116, 135, 143, 144, 176, 177, 185
Cleansers, face, 49, 50
  how to use, 49, 50
  deep pore, 50, 53
  medicated, 50, 56
  Directional Chart, 54
Clothing
  posture, 34
  walking, 37
  sitting, 39, 40
  putting on a coat, 42
  tanning, 57
  exercising, 111
  hairstyle, 120

INDEX

Clothing (*cont.*)
  color factors, 150–153
  fashion styles, 156–158
  classics and fads, 157, 158
  shopping skills, 158–160, 164
  use of line, 160
  body structure, 161, 162
  organizing wardrobe, 162–166
  wardrobe chart, 165
  basics, 166, 167
  accessories, 161, 162, 164, 168–174
  jewelry, 161, 164, 166, 168–170
  caring for, 174–176
  how to launder, 175, 176
  undergarments, 180
Color
  makeup, 62–67, 69–72
  hairstyle, 125, 126
  nails, 142, 143
  seasonal categories, 147, 148, color section
  skin tone, 148–150
  wardrobe, 150–153
  body type, 151
  effects, 151, 152
  redecorating a room, 152
  wheel, 152, 153, color section
  shopping tips, 159
Color Me Beautiful, 150
Combing, 42, 126, 130, 134
Conditioners, 118, 135
Confidence, 33, 42
  basis for, 23–25, 54, 61, 113, 147, 177, 193, 194
  and posture, 32–34
Contouring. *See* Face sculpting
Cooper, Wilhelmina, 18, 83, 187
Cosmetics. *See* Makeup
Creams, 49–51, 56, 63, 70, 111, 182, 183
Crossing (when seated)
  ankles, 40
  knees, 40
  legs, 40
Curling irons and brushes, 130

Dermatologist, consulting a, 50, 56, 58, 117
Designing Your Face, 62
Diet. *See* Nutrition
Dieting, 75, 76, 81, 82
  and exercise, 82, 91, 110, 111
Doors
  held open, 42, 43
  opening and closing, 43
Dress With Style, 150
Drugs, 76, 84, 85

Eating habits, 75–78, 80–82
  when exercising, 110, 111
  and hair, 135
Esther, Queen, 61

Exercises
  to improve posture, 34, 35
  to aid weight loss, 76, 78, 82, 84, 110
  and physical fitness, 91–113
  and hair, 119
Exfoliation, 50, 52, 54, 118, 181
Eye
  area care, 49–51, 53, 55, 57, 58, 64, 65, 172
  makeup, 49, 50, 65
  shadow, 49, 62, 66–68, 70, 72, 150, 152
  liner, 62, 66, 150
  lashes, 67
  lash curlers, 67
  brows, 67, 68
  color, 152

Face/facial
  expression, 34, 42, 177
  cleansing, 49, 50
  astringent, 50, 51
  moisturizer, 51, 52
  steaming, 52
  scrub, 52–54, 56
  masks, 50, 53, 54, 56
  Directional Chart, 54
  breakout, 55, 56
  shapes, 62, 63
  enhancement, 63, 64
  sculpting, 64, 65, 70
  and hairstyling, 120, 121
  waxing, 182
Feet, care of, 144, 181
  footwear, 171, 172
Figure. *See* Body
Fitness, physical, 91, 92
  aerobic exercises, 92–96
  nonaerobic exercises, 96, 97
  specific body areas, 98–108
  exercise chart, 109
  measurement chart, 110
  spiritual, 113, 114
Foundation, 48, 51, 52, 54, 57, 62–65, 70, 111
Freshener, 48, 51, 53

Gracefulness. *See* Posture; Visual poise
Gum chewing, 43

Hair
  health, 75, 119, 135
  structure, 116, 117
  basic care, 117, 118
  types of, 117, 123, 125
  trimming, 118, 119
  choosing a stylist, 119
  selecting a style, 119–121
  cuts, 121–123
  thinning, 122, 123
  chemical treatment, 125, 126
  tools and techniques, 126–131

INDEX

Hair (*cont.*)
   decorative styles, 131–133
   practical tips, 134, 135
   removing unwanted, 182, 183
Handbags, 41, 168, 170
Hands, 139, 143
   beauty tips, 144. *See also* Nails; Skin care
Hips, 36, 37, 97, 107, 110, 151, 161, 162

Jackson, Carole, 150

Lips
   makeup, 42, 49, 64, 70–72
   chapping, 51, 71
   and facial mask, 53
   color test, 70, 71, 150

Makeup, 42, 48–50, 53, 61–72, 120, 150, 153, color section
   and exercise, 111
Manicure, 139–142
Mascara, 50, 67, 72, 111
Masks
   facial, 50, 53, 54, 56
   spiritual, 54
Massaging, 117, 181, 182
Menstrual cycle, 55, 82, 110, 135, 181
Model's stance, 36, 38, 42
Moisturizer, 48, 50, 51, 53, 54, 56, 57, 71, 111
   tinted, 51
   after bath, 182
Mousse, 63, 118, 128, 130, 131

Nails, 71, 75
   care of, 139–142, 181
   repairing, 140, 143
   artificial, 143
   beauty tips, 143
Natural look, the, 63–67, 69–72, 153
Nutrition
   skin nourishment, 48, 55, 75
   hair, 75, 119, 135
   weight control, 76, 77, 81–84
   eating habits, 75, 77, 78, 80
   balanced food program, 78–80
   drugs and alcohol, 76, 84, 85
   spiritual diet, 85, 86
Nylons, 170, 171

Pedicure, 144
Perfume, 182–185
Permanents, 118, 125, 126
Picking up objects, 41
Pin curls, 130
Poise. *See* Visual poise
Posture
   importance of, 31, 32
   six points to perfect, 33, 34
   body alignment, 34
   exercises to improve, 34, 35
   standing, 35, 36
   walking, 36, 37
   turning around, 38
   sitting, 39, 40
   managing stairs, 40, 41
Powder, 64, 65, 69, 70, 72
   after bath, 182
Project pages
   healthy self-image, 26–28
   visual poise, 44, 45
   sensational skin, 59, 60
   model style makeup, 73
   nutrition, 87–89
   total fitness, 115
   hair happenings, 136, 137
   hands and nails, 145
   dazzle yourself with color, 154, 155
   functioning fashion, 178, 179
   delicate details, 186
   inner beauty, 195, 196
   self-image progress report, 198, 199
Purses, 41, 168, 170

Rinses, 118
Rollers, 128–130

Self-image, 16–25, 31, 32, 76. *See also* Confidence
Shaking hands, 42
Shampooing, 117, 118, 127, 135
Side-by-side stance, 35, 36
Sitting, 39, 40
Skin
   functions, 46, 47
   types, 47
   type test, 48
   nourishment, 48
   sunshine, 56–58
   exercise, 111
   color tone, 148–150
Skin breakout, 47, 50, 51, 55, 56, 64, 82, 111
Skin care
   diet, 48, 55, 75
   products, 48, 71
   basics, 49–52
   special techniques, 52–55, 181. *See also* Face; Exercises; Fitness, physical; Makeup; Nutrition; Skin breakout; Tanning
Smith, Jaclyn, 16
Split ends, 119, 126
Spotting, 38
Standing, 35, 36
Stippling, 64
Sun Protection Factor (SPF), 56–58
Sunburn, 58
Sunscreen, 56–58, 71

INDEX

Swayback, correcting, 35
Swimmer's hair, 118

T zone, 47
Tada, Joni Eareckson, 19
Tanning, 56
    do's and don'ts, 56–58
    self-tanning lotions, 58
Teeth, care of, 181
Toed-out toes, 37
Toner, 51
Turning in place, 38
Tweezing eyebrows, 68

Underarm protection, 182

Visual poise
    defined, 31

posture, 31–41
gracefulness, 29–31, 41–43
inner, 43

Walking, 34, 36, 37
    up and down stairs, 40, 41
    with escort, 42, 43
    and weight gain/loss, 81, 93
    for fitness, 93
Wallace, Joanne, 150
Wardrobe. *See* Clothing
Weight, 75–78
    gain, 81, 110
    loss, 82–84, 91, 93, 96, 110
Working Woman, The, 150

Yawning in public, 41, 42

INFORMATIONAL PAGE

I pray that the information in this book will get you started on the road to a more beautiful you—inside and out! Inner beauty far outweighs outer appearance, though we just can't let ourselves go ungroomed. A balanced combination will bring out the most attractive you!

If you are interested in having a Beautifully Created Seminar in your area, or would like information on Beautifully Created Summer Camp, please fill out the information below and return it to me.

Perhaps you have a question on one of the subjects covered in this book, or a problem you would like to share with me. Use the address below to contact me. I would be glad to write to you.

God bless you, and remember—because God created you and loves you, you can love yourself and be your best for Him.

My name is_____

My address is_____

City _____ State _____ Zip _____

Home phone (optional) (   )_____

I would like information on

_____ Beautifully Created Seminar

_____ Beautifully Created Summer Camp

_____ Cassette tape series

Mail to:
Beautifully Created
P.O. Box 1405
Santa Ynez, CA 93460